Environmental Health Criteria 87

ALLETHRINS — ALLETHRIN
d-ALLETHRIN
BIOALLETHRIN
S-BIOALLETHRIN

Published under the joint sponsorship of the United Nations Environment Programme, the International Labour Organisation, and the World Health Organization

World Health Organization
Geneva, 1989

The International Programme on Chemical Safety (IPCS) is a joint venture of the United Nations Environment Programme, the International Labour Organisation, and the World Health Organization. The main objective of the IPCS is to carry out and disseminate evaluations of the effects of chemicals on human health and the quality of the environment. Supporting activities include the development of epidemiological, experimental laboratory, and risk-assessment methods that could produce internationally comparable results, and the development of manpower in the field of toxicology. Other activities carried out by the IPCS include the development of know-how for coping with chemical accidents, coordination of laboratory testing and epidemiological studies, and promotion of research on the mechanisms of the biological action of chemicals.

ISBN 92 4 154287 X

The designations employed and the presentation of the material in this publication do not imply the expression of any opinion whatsoever on the part of the Secretariat of the World Health Organization concerning the legal status of any country, territory, city or area or of its authorities, or concerning the delimitation of its frontiers or boundaries.

The mention of specific companies or of certain manufacturers' products does not imply that they are endorsed or recommended by the World Health Organization in preference to others of a similar nature that are not mentioned. Errors and omissions excepted, the names of proprietary products are distinguished by initial capital letters.

PRINTED IN FINLAND

Vammalan Kirjapaino Oy

89/8039 — Vammala — 4500

CONTENTS

WHO TASK GROUP ON ENVIRONMENTAL HEALTH CRITERIA FOR ALLETHRINS AND RESMETHRINS

Members

Dr L.A. Albert-Palacios, National Institute of Biological Resources Research, Xalapa, Veracruz, Mexico[a]

Dr V. Benes, Institute of Hygiene and Epidemiology, Prague, Czechoslovakia

Dr A.H. El-Sabae, Faculty of Agriculture, Alexandria University, Alexandria, Egypt

Dr Y. Hayashi, National Institute of Hygienic Sciences, Tokyo, Japan

Dr S. Johnson, US Environmental Protection Agency, Hazard Evaluation Division, Washington DC, USA

Dr S.K. Kashyap, National Institute of Occupational Health, Ahmedabad, India (Vice-Chairman)

Dr J.H. Koeman, Agricultural University, Wageningen, Netherlands[a]

Dr Yu. I. Kundiev, Research Institute of Labour, Hygiene and Occupational Diseases, Kiev, USSR (Chairman)

Dr J.P. Leahey, ICI Agrochemicals Division, Jealotts Hill Research Station, Bracknell, Berkshire, United Kingdom (Rapporteur)

Dr M. Matsuo, Sumitomo Chemical Co. Ltd, Takarazuka Research Center, Takarazuka, Hyogo, Japan

Dr G.U. Oleru, College of Medicine, University of Lagos, Lagos, Nigeria

Observers

Mr J.-M. Pochon, International Group of National Associations of Agrochemical Manufacturers, Brussels, Belgium

Dr L.M. Sasynovitch, Research Institute of Hygiene and Toxicology of Pesticides, Polymers and Plastics, Kiev, USSR

---

[a] Invited but unable to attend.

Secretariat

Dr Z.P. Grigorevskaja, Centre for International Projects, Moscow, USSR

Dr K.W. Jager, International Programme on Chemical Safety, World Health Organization, Geneva, Switzerland (Secretary)

Dr J. Sekizawa, National Institute of Hygienic Sciences, Tokyo, Japan (Rapporteur)

NOTE TO READERS OF THE CRITERIA DOCUMENTS

Every effort has been made to present information in the criteria documents as accurately as possible without unduly delaying their publication. In the interest of all users of the environmental health criteria documents, readers are kindly requested to communicate any errors that may have occurred to the Manager of the International Programme on Chemical Safety, World Health Organization, Geneva, Switzerland, in order that they may be included in corrigenda, which will appear in subsequent volumes.

* * *

A detailed data profile and a legal file can be obtained from the International Register of Potentially Toxic Chemicals, Palais des Nations, 1211 Geneva 10, Switzerland (Telephone no. 988400 - 985850).

ENVIRONMENTAL HEALTH CRITERIA FOR ALLETHRINS

A WHO Task Group on Environmental Health Criteria for Allethrins and Resmethrins met in Moscow from 16-20 November 1987. The meeting was convened with the financial assistance of the United Nations Environment Programme (UNEP) and was hosted by the Centre for International Projects of the USSR State Committee on Science and Technology. On behalf of the USSR Commission for UNEP (UNEPCOM), Dr M. I. Gounar opened the Meeting and welcomed the participants. Dr K.W. Jager welcomed the participants on behalf of the Heads of the three IPCS cooperating organizations (UNEP/ILO/WHO). The Group reviewed and revised the draft Environmental Health Criteria and Health and Safety Guides and made an evaluation of the risks for human health and the environment from exposure to allethrins and resmethrins.

The first drafts of the documents were prepared by Dr J. Miyamoto and Dr M. Matsuo of Sumitomo Chemical Co. Ltd, with the assistance of the staff of the National Institute of Hygienic Sciences, Tokyo, Japan. Dr I. Yamamoto of the Tokyo University of Agriculture and Dr M. Eto of Kyushu University, Japan, assisted in the finalization of the draft.

The second draft was prepared by Dr J. Sekizawa of the National Institute of Hygienic Sciences, Tokyo, incorporating comments received following the circulation of the first draft to the IPCS contact points for Environmental Health Criteria documents.

The help of the Sumitomo Chemical Company Ltd, Japan and Roussel Uclaf, France in making their toxicological proprietary information on allethrins and resmethrins available to the IPCS and the Task Group is gratefully acknowledged. This enabled the Task Group to make their evaluation on a more complete data base.

The efforts of all who helped in the preparation and finalization of the documents are gratefully acknowledged.

* * *

Partial financial support for the publication of this criteria document was kindly provided by the United States Department of Health and Human Services, through a contract from the National Institute of Environmental Health Sciences, Research Triangle Park, North Carolina, USA - a WHO collaborating Centre for Environmental Health Effects. The United Nations Environment Programme (UNEP) generously supported the costs of printing.

* * *

<u>NOTE</u>: The proprietary information contained in this document cannot replace documentation for registration purposes, because the latter has to be closely linked to the source, the manufacturing route, and the purity/impurities of the substance to be registered. The data should be used in accordance with paragraphs 82-84 and recommendations paragraph 90 of the 2nd FAO Government Consultation (1982).

INTRODUCTION

SYNTHETIC PYRETHROIDS-A PROFILE

1. During investigations to modify the chemical structures of natural pyrethrins, a certain number of synthetic pyrethroids were produced with improved physical and chemical properties and greater biological activity. Several of the earlier synthetic pyrethroids were successfully commercialized, mainly for the control of household insects. Other more recent pyrethroids have been introduced as agricultural insecticides because of their excellent activity against a wide range of insect pests and their non-persistence in the environment.

2. The pyrethroids constitute another group of insecticides in addition to organochlorine, organophosphorus, carbamate, and other compounds. Pyrethroids commercially available to date include allethrin, resmethrin, d-phenothrin, and tetramethrin (for insects of public health importance), and cypermethrin, deltamethrin, fenvalerate, and permethrin (mainly for agricultural insects). Other pyrethroids are also available including furamethrin, kadethrin, and tellallethrin (usually for household insects), fenpropathrin, tralocythrin and tralomethrin, cyhalothrin, lambda-cyhalothrin, tefluthrin, cyfluthrin, flucythrinate, fluvalinate, and biphenate (for agricultural insects).

3. Toxicological evaluations of several synthetic pyrethroids have been performed by the FAO/WHO Joint Meeting on Pesticide Residues (JMPR). The acceptable daily intake (ADI) or temporary ADI has been estimated by the JMPR for cypermethrin, deltamethrin, fenvalerate, permethrin, phenothrin, cyfluthrin, cyhalothrin, and flucythrinate.

4. Chemically, synthetic pyrethroids are esters of specific acids (e.g., chrysanthemic acid, halo-substituted chrysanthemic acid, 2-(4-chlorophenyl)-3-methylbutyric acid) and alcohols (e.g., allethrolone, 3-phenoxybenzyl alcohol). For certain pyrethroids, the asymmetric centre(s) exist in the acid and/or alcohol moiety, and the commercial products sometimes consist of a mixture of both optical (1R/1S or d/l) and geometric (cis/trans)-isomers. However, most of the insecticidal activity of such products may reside in only one or two isomers. Some of the products (e.g., d-phenothrin, deltamethrin) consist only of such active isomer(s).

5. Synthetic pyrethroids are neuropoisons acting on the axons in the peripheral and central nervous systems by interacting with sodium channels in mammals and/or insects. A single dose produces toxic signs in mammals, such as tremors, hyperexcitability, salivation, choreoathetosis, and paralysis. The signs disappear fairly rapidly, and the animals recover, generally within a week. At near-lethal dose levels, synthetic pyrethroids cause transient changes in the nervous system, such as axonal swelling and/or breaks and myelin degeneration in sciatic nerves. They are not considered to cause delayed neurotoxicity of the kind induced by some organophosphorus compounds. The mechanism of toxicity of synthetic pyrethroids and their classification into two types are discussed in the Appendix.

6. Some pyrethroids (e.g., deltamethrin, fenvalerate, flucythrinate, and cypermethrin) may cause a transient itching and/or burning sensation in exposed human skin.

7. Synthetic pyrethroids are generally metabolized in mammals through ester hydrolysis, oxidation, and conjugation, and there is no tendency to accumulate in tissues. In the environment, synthetic pyrethroids are fairly rapidly degraded in soil and in plants. Ester hydrolysis and oxidation at various sites on the molecule are the major degradation processes. The pyrethroids are strongly adsorbed on soil and sediments, and hardly eluted with water. There is little tendency for bioaccumulation in organisms.

8. Because of low application rates and rapid degradation in the environment, residues in food are generally low.

9. Synthetic pyrethroids have been shown to be toxic for fish, aquatic arthropods, and honey-bees in laboratory tests. But, in practical usage, no serious adverse effects have been noticed, because of the low rates of application and lack of persistence in the environment. The toxicity of synthetic pyrethroids in birds and domestic animals is low.

10. In addition to the evaluation documents of FAO/WHO, there are several reviews and books on the chemistry, metabolism, mammalian toxicity, environmental effects, etc. of synthetic pyrethroids, including those by Elliot (1977), Miyamoto (1981), Miyamoto & Kearney (1983), and Leahey (1985).

1. SUMMARY

1.1 Identity, Physical and Chemical Properties, Analytical Methods

Allethrin was the first synthetic pyrethroid to be synthesized (in 1949) and was marketed in 1952. Chemically, it is an ester of chrysanthemic acid (CA), 2,2-dimethyl-3-(2,2-dimethylvinyl)cyclopropanecarboxylic acid with allethrolone and it is a racemic mixture of 8 stereoisomers: [1R,trans;1R]-, [1R,trans;1S]-, [1R,cis;1R]-, [1R,cis;1S]-, [1S,trans;1R]-, [1S,trans;1S]-, [1S,cis;1R]-, and [1S,cis;1S]-isomer. The ratio of the above isomers in the technical material is approximately 1:1:1:1:1:1:1:1. Among the isomers, the [1R,trans;1S]-isomer is the most biologically active followed by the [1R,cis;1S]-isomer. d-Allethrin consists of [1R,trans;1R]-, [1R,trans;1S]-, [1R,cis;1R]-, and [1R,cis;1S]-isomers in an approximate ratio of 4:4:1:1. Bioallethrin and esbiothrin consist of [1R,trans; 1R]- and [1R,trans;1S]-isomers. The isomeric composition of the former is approximately 1:1 and that of the latter, 1:3. S-Bioallethrin is the [1R,trans;1S]-isomer.

Allethrin is a clear, pale-yellow oil with a boiling point of 140 °C at a pressure of 0.1 mmHg; it is 75-95% pure. The specific gravity is 1.005 at 25 °C. Allethrin is practically insoluble in water, but soluble in organic solvents, such as methanol, hexane, and xylene. It is unstable in light, air, and under alkaline conditions. It is decomposed by rapid pyrolysis at over 400 °C, but vaporizes without decomposing, when heated at 150 °C. It is fairly volatile.

d-Allethrin is an oily liquid (specific gravity of 1.005-1.015 at 20 °C).

Bioallethrin is an amber-coloured, viscous liquid.

Esbiothrin is a yellow, viscous liquid.

S-Bioallethrin is a yellow liquid.

Allethrin residues and levels in environmental samples are determined by dual-wavelength densitometry (370 or 230 nm), or by derivatisation and colorimetric measurement at levels as low as 0.1 mg/litre. A gas chromatograph with flame ionization detector is used for analysis of the technical product.

1.2 Production and Uses

It is estimated that several hundred tonnes of allethrin, d-allethrin, bioallethrin, esbiothrin, and S-Bioallethrin are manufactured and used yearly throughout the world, mainly for the control of household insects. Formulations include aerosol sprays, smoke coils, electric mats, and emulsifiable concentrates, with or without synergists or other insecticides.

1.3 Residues in Food

No information is available on the levels of allethrin residues in treated crops. Allethrin was not detected in the milk of dairy cows or in the meat of a female goat, which had been sprayed daily for 3 and 5 weeks, respectively (limit of detection of method used - 0.1 mg/kg).

1.4 Environmental Fate

The photodegradation rate was measured of a thin film of allethrin on glass under a sun lamp. Approximately 8 h of exposure were needed for 90% degradation. S-Bioallethrin was rapidly decomposed, when similarly exposed to sunlight. The major photoreactions were ester cleavage, di-π-methane rearrangement, oxidation at the isobutenyl methyl group, epoxidation at the isobutenyl double bond, and cis/trans-isomerization. The major degradation products formed were CA, the 3-(2-hydroxymethyl) or the 3-(1-epoxy) derivative of allethrin, and cyclopropylrethronyl chrysanthemate. Sunlight photolysis of allethrin in solution yielded similar products. Allethrin was decomposed by rapid pyrolysis at over 400 °C. When kept at 150 °C for 9 h in an aluminum foil vessel in air, it vaporized (28-35%), polymerized (24-45%), and decomposed (18-40%). CA, allethrolone, pyrocin, and cis-dihydrochrysanthemo-δ-lactone were the degradation products formed.

1.5 Kinetics and metabolism

When ^{14}C-acid- or ^{3}H-alcohol-labelled allethrin was administered orally to rats at a rate of 1-5 mg/kg body weight, the radiocarbon and tritium were eliminated in the urine (30% and 20.7%, respectively) and faeces (29% and 27%, respectively) within 48 h. The major metabolic reactions were ester hydrolysis, oxidation at the trans-methyl of the isobutenyl group, gem-dimethyl of the cyclopropane ring, and the methylene of the allyl group, and 2,3-diol formation at the allylic group. The major urinary metabolites were chrysanthemum dicarboxylic acid, allethrolone, and some oxidized forms of allethrin.

1.6 Effects on Experimental Animals and In Vitro Test Systems

The acute oral toxicities of all the allethrins are weak to moderate with LD_{50} values ranging from 210 mg/kg body weight (mouse) to 4290 mg/kg (rabbit). On the basis of limited data, the dermal toxicity appears to be very low (LD_{50} > 2000 mg/kg for the rabbit). The inhalation toxicity values (LC_{50} values) for the allethrins were found to be > 1500 mg/m^3 (in the mouse and rat).

Allethrin is a Type I pyrethroid. The Type I syndrome involves hyperactivity, tremors, convulsion, and paralysis in mammals and insects (see Appendix).

Bioallethrin and esbiothrin are classified as compounds producing mild primary irritation of the skin of New Zealand White rabbits and slight irritation of the eyes.

When a 10% olive oil solution of allethrin was applied to the eyes of rabbits, slight hyperaemia of the conjunctiva and eye discharge were observed 10 min and 2 h after application, respectively.

When a 5% olive oil solution of allethrin was applied to the skin of guinea-pigs, every other day, 10 times in all, and animals were challenged with an intradermal injection 2 weeks after the last application, there was no sensitization reaction, but slight lymphocytic and monocytic infiltration of the dermis was noted.

No adverse reactions were observed when the primary dermal irritancy of S-Bioallethrin was evaluated in Wistar rats and Nagano white rabbits.

When rats were fed allethrin in the diet at dose levels of up to 10 000 mg/kg for 16 weeks, tremor and convulsions were noted at 10 000 mg/kg, but no gross effects were seen at 5000 mg/kg.

Allethrin was administered orally, using a syringe, to rats at dose levels of up to 1000 mg/kg body weight per day, once a day, 6 days a week for 12 weeks. Half of the rats died following a single administration of 1000 mg/kg. Higher relative weights of the liver, thyroid, and kidney were noted at lower doses.

Inhalation of allethrin by mice at a level of 3 g/m^3 for 4 h a day, 6 days a week, over 4 weeks, resulted in eye discharge in all animals. Histopathological examination of the lungs revealed bronchopneumonia.

S-Bioallethrin was also tested via the inhalation route in several studies conducted on mice and rats at a range of dose levels (10, 20, or 25 times the normal concentration used) for exposure periods of up to 5 weeks. The results of these studies indicated that the short-term toxicity of S-Bioallethrin is low.

Bioallethrin was administered in the diet to rats for 90 days at levels of 500, 1500, 5000, or 10 000 mg/kg. Slight or moderate decreases in body weight gain and slight liver dysfunction were found at the 5000 and 10 000 mg/kg levels. A no-observed-adverse-effect level of 1500 mg/kg was determined.

When the same compound was administered in the diet of dogs, for 6 months, at levels of 200, 1000, or 5000 mg/kg, general body trembling, irregular heart rhythm, and increases in the mean levels of alkaline phosphatase and SGPT were noted at the 5000 mg/kg level. Hepatocellular degeneration was found at both the 1000 and 5000 mg/kg levels. A no-observed-adverse-effect level of 200 mg/kg was established.

F344 rats were administered d-allethrin at levels of 0, 125, 500, or 2000 mg/kg diet for 123 weeks. Decreased body weight and hepatotoxic effects were observed at levels exceeding 500 mg/kg diet (i.e., 24.5 mg/kg body weight per day). However, no oncogenic effects were observed at any dose and the no-observed-adverse-effect level was 5.9 mg/kg body weight per day.

Dogs were fed allethrin at a rate of 50 mg/kg body weight per day for 2 years. There were no compound-related gross or microscopic changes at this level.

Allethrin, bioallethrin, esbiothrin, and S-Bioallethrin have been evaluated in a variety of mutagenicity tests, including *in vitro*/*in vivo* gene mutation, DNA damage and repair, and *in vitro*/*in vivo* chromosomal aberrations. The results of all studies were assessed as negative.

Allethrin, bioallethrin, and S-Bioallethrin were tested for embryotoxicity and teratogenicity in rats, mice, and rabbits. No compound-related embryo toxicity or teratogenicity were observed in these studies, though some variations were observed in some studies.

S-Bioallethrin did not seem to induce any disorders in the fetuses of pregnant Wistar rats at doses of 100 mg/kg per day, or less. Furthermore, S-Bioallethrin did not induce any teratogenic effects in the pregnant TVCS mice at the maximum tolerated dose of 100 mg/kg per day.

Allethrin was administered daily in corn oil, by gavage, at doses of 0, 215, or 350 mg/kg body weight to pregnant albino rabbits from day 6 to day 18 of gestation. No fetotoxic or teratogenic effects were observed.

1.7 Effects on Organisms in the Environment

Allethrin, bioallethrin, and S-Bioallethrin are all toxic for fish with LC_{50} values of 9-90 µg/litre, S-Bioallethrin being the most toxic. Allethrin is generally less toxic for *Daphnia* and aquatic insect larvae with LC_{50} values of 150-50 000 µg/litre.

The toxicity of allethrin is low for birds (LD_{50} > 2000 mg/kg), but high for honey-bees (LD_{50} 3-9 µg/bee).

2. IDENTITY, PHYSICAL AND CHEMICAL PROPERTIES, ANALYTICAL METHODS

2.1 Identity

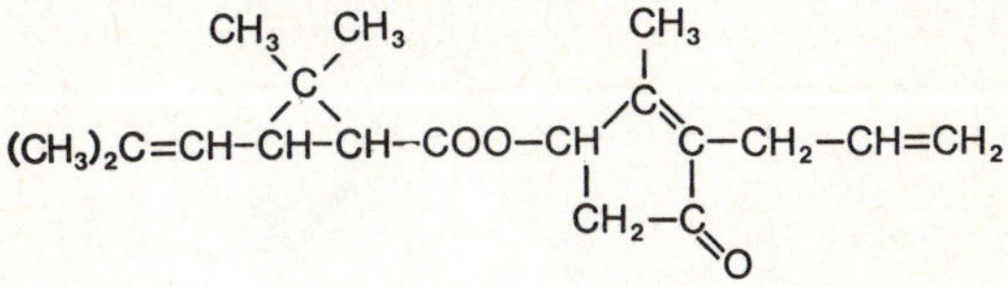

Allethrin, the first of the synthetic pyrethroids, was discovered by Schechter et al. (1949), when simplifying the chemical structures of natural pyrethrins. It is a mixture of 8 stereo isomers (Fig. 1) and is less volatile and more stable to heat and light than the natural pyrethrins.

The 3S:3R or cis:trans ratio is reported to be 1:1 and the optical ratio of 1R:1S in the acid and allethronyl moiety is also 1:1 (racemic). Technical grade material contains 75-95% allethrin. d-Allethrin is the ester of the (1R, cis, trans)-acid with racemic allethrolone. Bioallethrin and esbiothrin are the (1R,trans)-acid ester of racemic allethrolone. S-Bioallethrin is the ester of the (1R,trans)-acid with (1S)-allethrolone. The compositions of these isomers are shown in Table 1.

The technical product (Esbiol) contains 90% S-Bioallethrin.

2.2 Physical and Chemical Properties

Some physical and chemical properties of allethrins are given in Table 2.

Data on melting points were not available. Allethrin is unstable to light and air and under alkaline conditions. However, it is more stable on exposure to heat and light than pyrethrins. Allethrin is decomposed by rapid pyrolysis at over 400 °C, but vaporizes without decomposition (28-35%) when heated at 150 °C. d-Allethrin is soluble in most organic solvents. d-Allethrin, bioallethrin, and S-Bioallethrin are also unstable to light, in air, and under alkaline conditions. S-Bioallethrin is miscible with most organic solvents (FAO/WHO, 1965; Martin & Worthing, 1977; Meister et al., 1983; Worthing & Walker, 1983; Devaux & Bolla, 1986a,b; Devaux & Tillier, 1986).

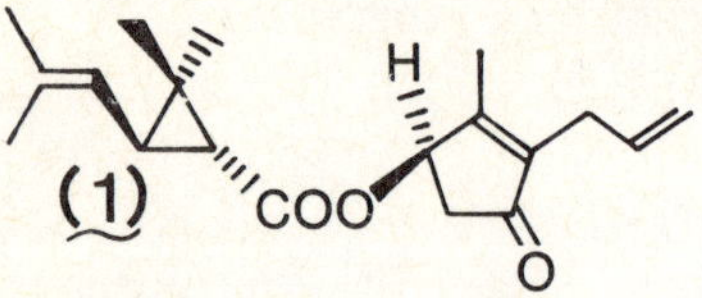

(1) (1R,trans) (1R)

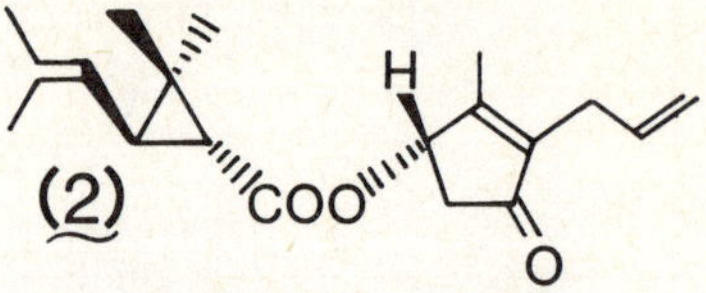

(2) (1R,trans) (1S)

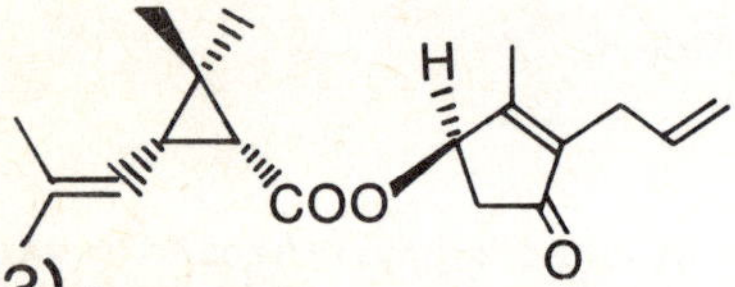

(3) (1R,cis) (1R)

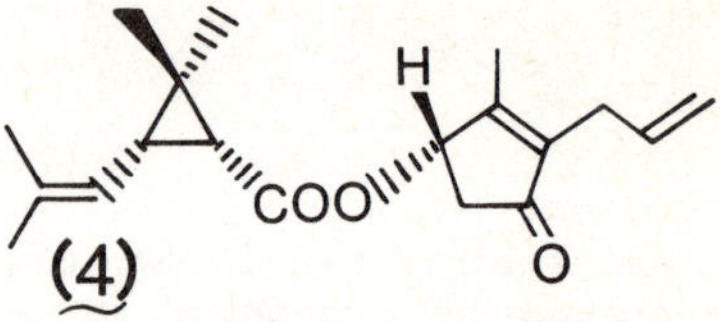

(4) (1R.cis) (1S)

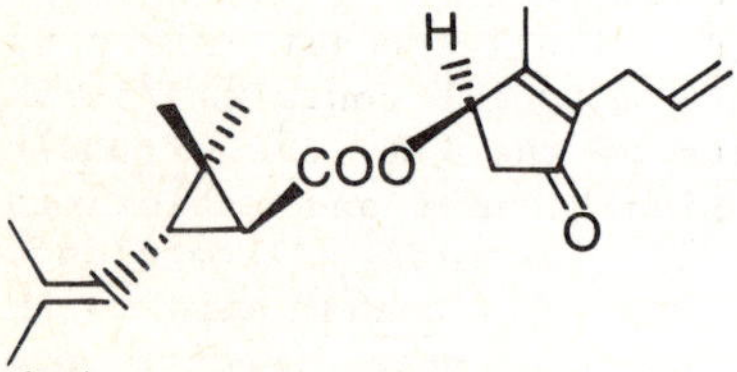

(5) (1S,trans) (1R)

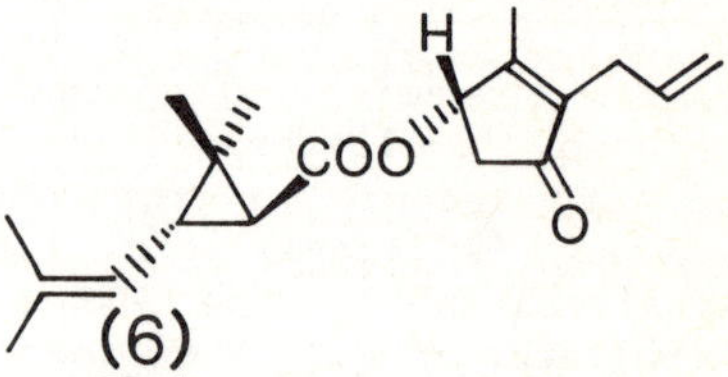

(6) (1S,trans) (1S)

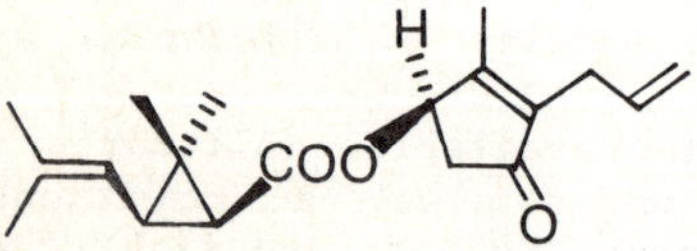

(7) (1S,cis) (1R)

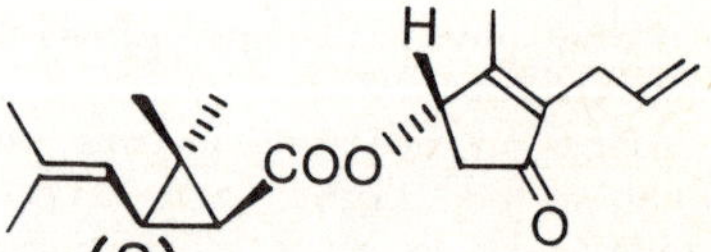

(8) (1S,cis) (1S)

Fig. 1. Chemical structures of 8 stereoisomers.

Table 1. Chemical identity of allethrins of various stereoisomeric compositions

Common name/ CAS Registry No./ NIOSH Accession No.[a]	CA Index name (9CI) Stereospecific name[b,c]	Stereoisomeric composition[d]	Synonyms and trade names
Allethrin[e] 584-79-2[f] GZ1476000	2-methyl-4-oxo-3-(2-propenyl)-2-cyclopenten-1-yl 2,2-dimethyl 3-(2-methyl-1-propenyl) cyclopropanecarboxylate (9CL) (RS)-3-Allyl-2-methyl-4-oxocyclopent-2-enyl (1RS, *cis*, *trans*)-2,2-dimethyl-3-(2,2-dimethylvinyl)cyclopropanecarboxylate or (RS)-Allethronyl (1RS, *cis*, *trans*)-chrysanthemate	(1):(2):(3):(4):(5):(6):(7):(8)=1:1:1:1:1:1:1:1	Pallethrin, Pynamin, Allycinerin, Pyresin, Pyresyn, Necarboxylic acid, ENT17,510, FDA1446, FMC249, NIA249, RU 28173 Allethrin concentrate MGK
d-Allethrin	same as allethrin (RS)-Allethronyl [1R, *cis*, *trans*]-chrysanthemate	(1):(2):(3):(4)=4:4:1:1	d-*cis*, *trans*-Allethrin Pynamin Forte
Bioallethrin 584-79-2[f] GZ1950000	same as allethrin (RS)-Allethronyl [1R, *trans*]-chrysanthemate	(1):(2)=1:1	d-*trans*-Allethrin (+)-*trans*-Allethrin RU 11705 Depallethrin
Esbiothrin	same as allethrin (RS)-Allethronyl [1R, *trans*]-chrysanthemate	(1):(2)=1:3	RU 27436

Table 1 (contd).

Common name/ CAS Registry No./ NIOSH Accession No.[a]	CA Index name (9CI) / Stereospecific name[b,c]	Stereoisomeric composition[d]	Synonyms and trade names
S-Bioallethrin 28434-00-6 GZ1472000	same as allethrin (S)-Allethronyl [1R, *trans*]-chrysanthemate	(2)	Esbiol, Esdepallethrin d-Allethronyl d-*trans* allethrin (+)-Allethronyl (+)-*trans*-allethrin RU 16121
- - GZ1460000	same as allethrin (RS)-Allethronyl [1R, *cis*]-chrysanthemate	-	d-*cis*-Allethrin (+)-*cis*-Allethrin
- - GZ1925000	same as allethrin (S)-Allethronyl [1R, *cis*, *trans*]-chrysanthemate	-	-

a NIOSH (1983).
b (1R), d, (+) or (1S), 1, (-) in the acid part of allethrin signifies the same stereospecific conformation, respectively. (S), d, (+) or (R), 1, (-) in the alcohol part of allethrin signify the same stereospecific conformation, respectively.
c Allethronyl radical is a name of the radical that forms the alcohol part of allethrin. Chrysanthemic acid is a name of the acid that forms the acid part of allethrin.
d Numbers in parentheses identify the structures shown in the figures of stereoisomers.
e ISO common name: common names for pesticides and other agrochemicals approved by the Technical Committee of the International Organization for Standardization.
f CAS Registry No. 584-79-2 is assigned to both allethrin and bioallethrin.

Table 2. Physical and chemical properties of allethrins

	Allethrin	d-Allethrin	Bio-allethrin	Esbiothrin	S-Bio-allethrin
Physical state	oil	oily liquid	viscous liquid	viscous liquid	liquid
Colour	pale yellow	-	amber	yellow	yellow
Odour	-	-	aromatic	-	-
Relative molecular mass	302.45	302.45	302.45	302.45	302.45
Boiling point (°C)	140 (0.1 mmHg)	-	153 (0.4mmHg)	-	-
Flash point (°C)	-	130	65.6	-	-
Solubility in water	low	low	low[a]	low	low
Solubility in organic solvents	soluble[b]	soluble	soluble[c]	soluble	soluble
Density	d^{25}_{4} 1.005	d^{20}_{4} 1.005 - 1.015	d^{20}_{4} 0.997	-	d^{20}_{4} 0.980
Vapour pressure	1.2×10^{-4} mmHg (30 °C)	-	3.3×10^{-4} mmHg (25 °C)	-	-
n-Octanol/water partition coefficient	-	-	4.8×10^{4} (25 °C)	-	-

a 4.6 mg/litre at 25 °C.
b Methanol (> 1 kg/kg), hexane (> 1kg/kg), xylene (> 1kg/kg), acetone, carbon tetrachloride, kerosene, petroleum.
c Acetone, ethanol, hexane, methylene chloride, kerosene.

2.3 Analytical Methods

A limited number of publications is available on methods of analysis for allethrin residues and analysis of environmental media. Analytical procedures listed in Table 3 include (a) extraction with solvent, (b) partition, (c) clean up, (d) suitable analytical instruments and conditions, and (e) minimum detectable concentration and recovery for each method.

The stereoselectivity of a radioimmunoassay (RIA) system using an S-Bioallethrin-specific antiserum was studied by observing the abilities of the 8 allethrin isomers and other selected compounds to compete with a radiolabelled S-Bioallethrin tyramine derivative for antibody-binding sites (Wing & Hammock, 1979). The results demonstrate the feasibility of RIA as a rapid, sensitive, and stereoselective residue technique for compounds difficult to analyse using classical methods.

Table 3. Analytical methods for allethrin[a]

Sample	Sample preparation			Determination		Limit of detection (mg/litre)	% Recovery (fortification) (mg/litre)	Reference
	Extraction solvent	Partition	Clean-up method	Derivatization	Detection method			
Analysis for Residues								
Milk Meat	petroleum ether			mercuric oxide/ sulfuric acid	colorimetric	0.1		McClellan & Moore (1958)
Wheat	petroleum spirit			modified Deniges reagent	colorimetric (584 nm)			Desmarchelier (1976)
Analysis for total content								
Dish Apple Spinach (dislodgeable residue)	n-hexane	n-hexane/ CH_3CN	HPTLC benzene/ CCl_4 (1 + 1) n-hexane/ether/ formic acid (70/30/1)		dual-wavelength densitometry (1 = 370 nm; 2 = 230 nm)		91-104% (300 µg) 98% (300 µg) 92% (300 µg)	Uno et al. (1982)
Mosquito coil	toluene +99% formic acid (5:1)				FID-GC		94-102%	Sakaue et al. (1985)

Table 3 (contd).

Sample	Sample preparation			Determination		Limit of detection (mg/litre)	% Recovery (fortification) (mg/litre)	Reference
	Extraction solvent	Partition	Clean-up method	Derivatization	Detection method			
Product analysis								
Technical grade	acetone				FID-GC, N_2 40 ml/min, 1 m; 5% DEGS, 180 °C, 8.4 min			Murano (1972)

a FID = Flame ionization detector; GC = gas chromatography; UV = ultraviolet; HPTLC = high-performance thin-layer chromatography.

3. SOURCES IN THE ENVIRONMENT, ENVIRONMENTAL TRANSPORT, DISTRIBUTION AND TRANSFORMATION, ENVIRONMENTAL LEVELS AND HUMAN EXPOSURE

3.1 Industrial Production

Allethrin is prepared by the esterification of [1RS, 3RS or cis, trans]-2,2-dimethyl-3-(2,2-dimethylvinyl) cyclopropanecarboxylic acid or chrysanthemic acid with (1RS)-3-allyl-2-methyl-4-oxocyclopent-2-ene-1-ol or allethrolone (Sanders & Taff, 1954).

It was first marketed in 1952, in Japan and the USA (Yoshioka, 1980). At present, several hundred tonnes are thought to be manufactured annually throughout the world, mainly for the control of household insect pests. Bioallethrin was first marketed in early 1970 and is now used at a rate of 10 - 30 tonnes per year. Formulations of allethrin combined with organophosphorus insecticides, such as tetrachlorvinphos and fenitrothion, are produced for agricultural use (Japan Plant Protection Association, 1984).

3.2 Use Patterns

Allethrin is used mainly for the control of flies and mosquitoes in the home, flying and crawling insects on farm animals, and fleas and ticks on dogs and cats. It is formulated as aerosols (1-6 g/litre), sprays, dusts (1%), smoke coils, and mats. It is used alone or combined with synergists (e.g., piperonyl butoxide and N-octylbicycloheptene dicarboximide) or other insecticides (e.g., fenitrothion). It is also available in the form of emulsifiable concentrates (810 g/kg) and wettable powders. Synergistic formulations (aerosols or dips) have been used on fruits and berries, post-harvest, in storage, and in processing plants. Post-harvest use on stored grain (surface treatment) has also been approved in some countries (FAO/WHO 1965). No information is available on recent post-harvest treatment with allethrin.

Bioallethrin is more than twice as effective as allethrin and is mainly used to control household insects. It is formulated as aerosols and sprays with synergists and/or other insecticides (e.g., d-phenothrin or deltamethrin). A few tonnes of bioallethrin have been used in Spain for this purpose, according to Battelle (1982). Since 1982, this aerosol formulation has been used in many other countries. The use of mosquito coils and electric mats has also increased considerably.

S-Bioallethrin is several times as effective as allethrin against flying and crawling insects and is mainly used in industry and in the home. It is formulated as aerosols and sprays with synergists for use as a knock-down or flushing agent. Several tonnes of S-Bioallethrin were used for this purpose in 1980 in France, together with bioallethrin and allethrin (Battelle, 1982).

3.3 Environmental Transport, Distribution, and Transformation

Degradation pathways of allethrin are summarized in Fig. 2.

When exposed as a thin film or coating on glass (2.6 µg/cm²) to a sunlamp for 8 h, [^{14}C]-trans-allethrin was rapidly decomposed to give at least 14 products. The photoproducts derived from the carboxy (acid) - and allethrolone (alcohol) - labelled compounds showed a similar TLC pattern, indicating that most, if not all, of the products were esters. Saponification of the mixture of esters liberated 16 acids including trans-carbonic acid and keto derivatives arising from the oxidative attack at the double bond of the isobutenyl moiety, and chrysanthemic acid derivatives having the trans-methyl in the isobutenyl side chain oxidized to the alcohol, aldehyde and carboxylic acid. There was no cis/trans-isomerization, even after extended irradiation for up to 24 h (Chen & Casida, 1969).

The photodegradation rates of a thin film (54 µg/cm²) under a sunlamp were compared for trans-allethrin, pyrethrin-I, tetramethrin, and dimethrin. The rates of transformation varied dramatically with variation in the alcohol moieties, and the exposure times needed for 90% loss of the original compound were approximately 0.2, 4, 8, and 16 h, for pyrethrin-I, tetramethrin, allethrin, and dimethrin, respectively. The chemical reactions involved in the alcohol moieties were not clarified (Chen & Casida, 1969).

The photostability under sunlight of bioallethrin included in, or mixed with, beta-cyclodextrin was studied. Inclusion slowed down the decomposition of allethrin, the half-life extending from 3 days for the free state to about 35 days for the included form. Inclusion retarded the photochemical decomposition of the acid moiety, compared with the alcohol moiety (Yamamoto et al., 1976).

Irradiation of a diastereomer mixture of bioallethrin in hexane or kerosene, using a medium or high pressure mercury arc lamp, resulted in the formation of the cyclopropylrethronyl chrysanthemates (13,15 in Fig. 2) (approx. 90%) via di-π-methane rearrangement at the allyl substituent in the alcohol moiety (Fig. 2). The same product was formed in kerosene and in sunlight. The reaction was completely

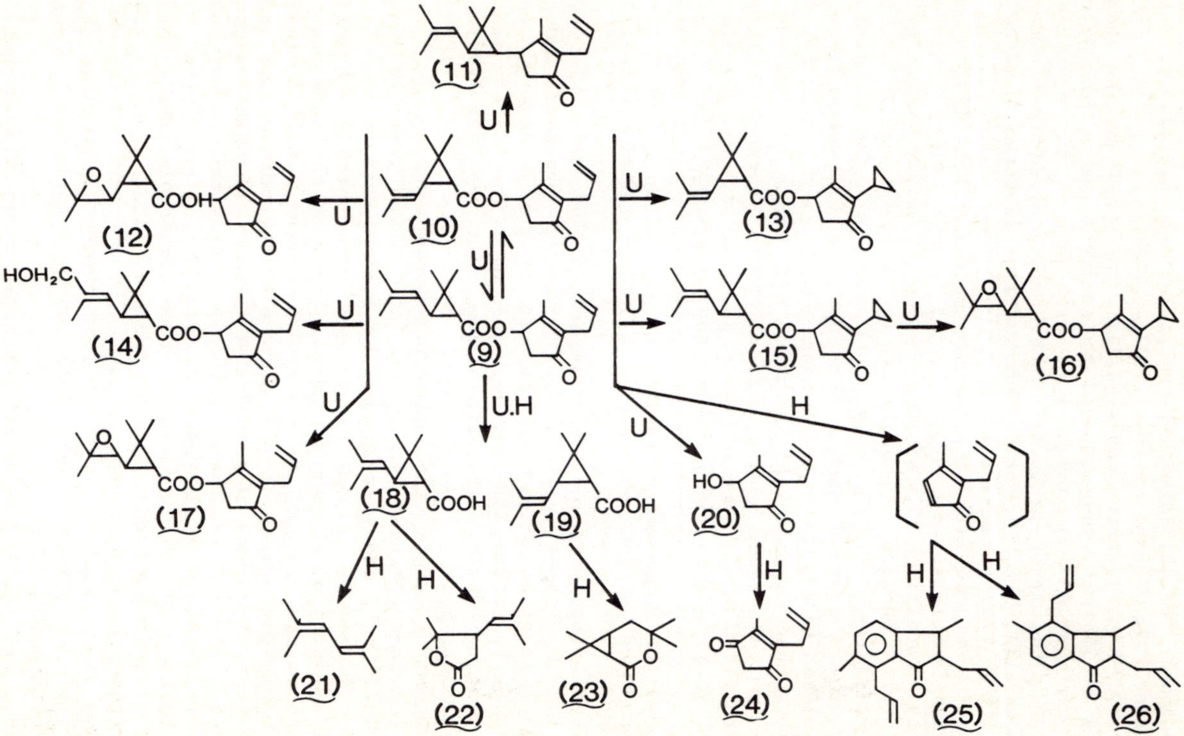

Fig. 2. Degradation pathways of allethrin by UV radiation and heat
(U = UV radiation; H = heat).

quenched by 2,5-dimethylhexa-2,4-diene. No evidence was obtained of the accompanying formation of either cis-cyclopropane- or 3,3-dimethylacrylic esters (Bullivalent & Pattenden, 1973; Kawano et al., 1980).

S-[^{14}C]-Bioallethrin labelled in the acid moiety was rapidly decomposed, when exposed to sunlight as a thin film (25 μg/cm^2) on glass. After 3 h, with 56% of the compound converted, the major products identified resulted from ester cleavage (18) (14.7%), oxidation at the isobutenyl methyl group (14) (7.9%), di-π-methane rearrangement (15) (9.9%), epoxidation at the isobutenyl double bond (16,17) (16%), and cis/trans-isomerization (10) (1.2%). Many minor photoproducts, totalling 55% of the reaction mixture, were not identified. Sunlight photolysis in solution (1.8-7.2 X 10^{-3} mol/litre) for 3 h yielded most of the products observed in the solid phase. More epoxides (17) were formed in benzene (33%) than in hexane (12%), and in aerated solutions than in solutions saturated with argon or nitrogen. In acetonitrile-water (4:1), S-Bioallethrin reacted to form cyclopropylrethronyl chrysanthemate (15) (70%), a cis/trans-isomerization product (10) (14%), and epoxides (17) (8%) in the acid moiety. Formation of chrysanthemic acid (18) by ester bond cleavage was comparable in all solvents (4-6%) but was increased in the presence of a benzil radical (Ruzo et al., 1980).

Direct photolysis of S-Bioallethrin in benzene under UV radiation (360 nm) yielded the products observed under sunlight, together with trace amounts of the decarboxylated derivative (11), the cis-epoxides, and more than twenty-five other minor products. Triplet intermediates were involved in the cyclopropane isomerization and the di-π-methane rearrangement, since the reactions were enhanced by a sensitizer benzophenone, especially at a high concentration (0.1 mol/litre), and were blocked by 1,3-cyclohexadiene. The epoxides formed by triplet oxygen were considerably enhanced by the addition of a benzil radical, and were the only major products in the presence of 1,3-cyclohexadiene. Oxidation at the trans-methyl group in the chrysanthemate moiety resulted from radical reactions of ground-state oxygen. Singlet oxygen was not involved in these oxidation reactions since the sensitizer, Rose Bengal, gave a totally different product distribution under UV radiation. Under comparable conditions, the cyclopropylrethronyl chrysanthemate (15), formed via di-π-methane rearrangement, reacted in benzene under UVR (360 nm) more slowly than the parent compound, yielding the corresponding epoxides (16) (15%) and allethrin (9) (70%) (Ruzo et al., 1980).

The rapid pyrolysis of allethrin and other chrysanthemic esters was examined by gas-liquid chromatography (GLC) with a sample injection port heated at 250-550 °C. Allethrin was less stable than any of the other compounds, including tetramethrin, at temperatures of over 400 °C, because of the instability of the allethrolone moiety (Kyogoku et al., 1970).

Allethrin in a pyrex glass tube heated at 400 °C, under nitrogen, gave chrysanthemic acid, 2,6-dimethylhepta-2,4-diene (21) and pyrocin (22) as pyrolysis products from the acid moiety, and 2,7-diallyl-3,6-dimethyl-1-indanone (25) and 2,4-diallyl-3,5-dimethyl-1-indanone (26) from the alcohol moiety (Nakada et al., 1971).

Baba & Ohno (1972) studied the vaporization and degradation of allethrin (100 mg) in an aluminum foil vessel in air at 150 °C for 9 h. Under these conditions, 28-35% of allethrin vaporized without undergoing any changes, 24-45% polymerized, and 18-40% decomposed. The thermal degradation products formed were trans-chrysanthemic acid (18) and allethrolone (20), together with 2-allyl-3-methylcyclopenta-2-ene-1,4-dione (24), which was formed by subsequent pyrolysis of allethrolone. In addition, cis-chrysanthemic acid (19), pyrocin (22), and cis-dihydrochrysanthemo-δ-lactone (23) were formed under the same conditions from the mixture of 8 isomers of allethrin; cis-dihydroxy-chrysanthemo-δ-lactone (23) was produced from cis-allethrin.

3.4 Environmental Levels and Human Exposure

No information is available on levels of allethrins in the environment or on general population or occupational levels of exposure.

3.4.1 Residues in food

No information is available on the levels of allethrin residues in treated crops. Allethrin was not detected (detection limit 0.1 mg/kg) in the milk of dairy cows that had been sprayed daily for 3 weeks or in the meat tissue of a female goat that had been sprayed daily for 5 weeks, all animals receiving a large overdose of spray. No information is available on the chemical nature of the terminal residues in treated crops (FAO/WHO, 1965).

4. KINETICS AND METABOLISM

4.1 Metabolism in Mammals

Metabolic pathways of allethrin in mammals are summarized in Fig. 3.

When allethrin (9) labelled with ^{14}C in the acid moiety or with ^{3}H in the alcohol moiety was administered orally to male Sprague Dawley rats at levels ranging from 1 to 5 mg/kg body weight, the radiocarbon and tritium from the acid- and alcohol-labellings were eliminated in the urine (30% and 20.7%, respectively) and faeces (29% and 27%, respectively) in 48 h. The tissue residues were not determined. Most of the metabolites excreted in the urine were ester-form metabolites together with two hydrolysed products, chrysanthemum dicarboxylic acid (29) (CDCA) and allethrolone (20). The faecal metabolites were not identified. Allethrin could have been metabolized via any of the following 5 biotransformation pathways; hydrolysis to allethrolone and to a smaller extent CDCA, formation of the 2,3-diol (30) from the allyl moiety, hydroxylation at the methylene position of the allyl grouping (31), hydroxylation at one of the geminal dimethyl groups (32), and oxidation at the trans methyl group of the isobutenyl moiety to carboxylic acid (28) (Elliott et al., 1972a,b; Yamamoto, 1970).

4.2 Enzymatic Systems for Biotransformation

The microsome or microsome-plus-soluble fraction prepared from rat or mouse liver homogenate was incubated in a phosphate buffer (0.1 mol/litre, pH 7.4) for 30 min at 37 °C with 7 or 70 µg allethrin, in the presence or absence of NADPH. Allethrin yielded neutral metabolites (ex. 14, 27), several acidic metabolites (ex. 28, 29), and some other polar metabolites, when examined using two-dimensional thin-layer chromatography (Elliot et al., 1972a,b).

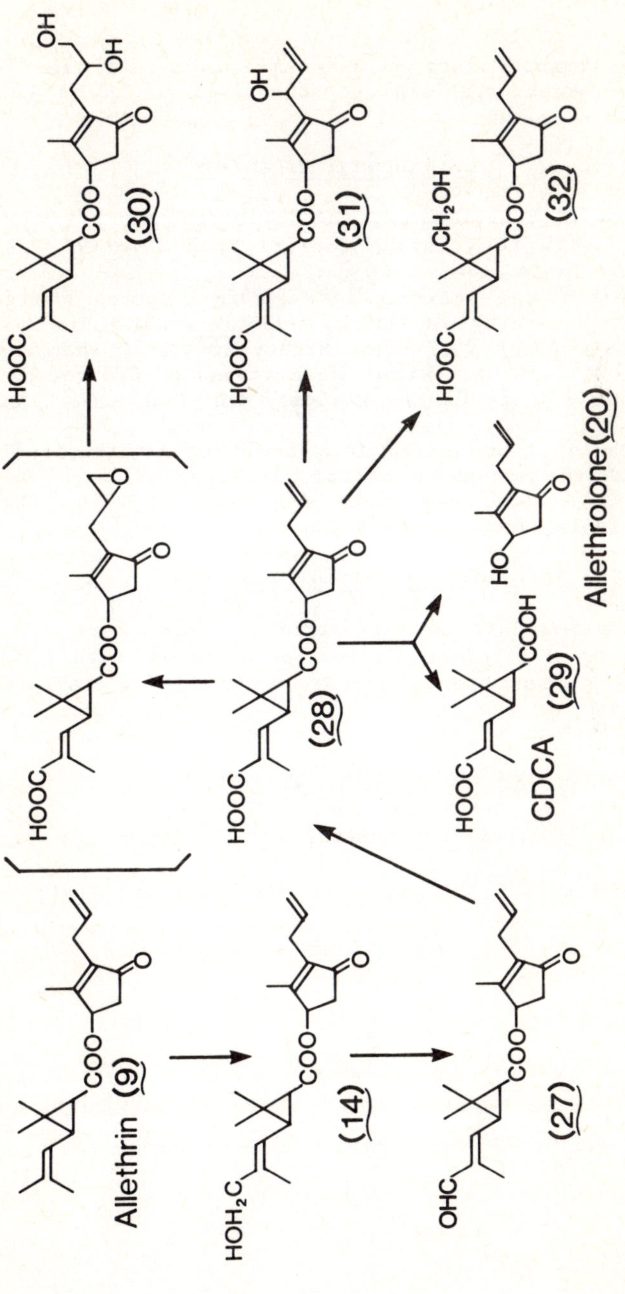

Fig. 3. Metabolic pathways of allethrin in mammals.

5. EFFECTS ON ORGANISMS IN THE ENVIRONMENT

Acute toxicity data on allethrin in aquatic and terrestrial non-target organisms are summarized in Tables 4 and 5, respectively.

5.1 Aquatic Organisms

Allethrin, bioallethrin, and S-Bioallethrin are all toxic for fish, with LC_{50} values ranging from 9 to 90 µg/litre, as shown in Table 4.

The biological activity in fish is affected by temperature. The toxicity of 1R or (+)-*trans*-allethrin for the bluegill was about 1.5 times higher at 22 °C than at 12 °C (Mauck et al., 1976). Water hardness and pH did not have any significant effects on the toxicity for fish (Mauck et al., 1976).

Allethrin is generally less toxic in arthropods than in fish, with the exception of the stonefly, which is the most susceptible insect, having a 96-h LC_{50} of 2 µg/litre, as shown in Table 4.

5.2 Terrestrial Organisms

Only a few data on terrestrial organisms are available. The toxicity of allethrin is low for birds and high for honeybees, as has been observed for other pyrethroids (Table 5).

Table 4. Acute toxicity of allethrin for non-target aquatic organisms

Species	Size	Parameter	Concentration (µg/litre)	Formulation[a]	System	Temperature (°C)	pH	Hardness (mg $CaCO_3$/litre) or salinity (%)	Reference
Fish									
Salmon (Salmo salar)	10 cm; 11.07 g	96-h LC_{50}	16.5	technical	renewal	10			Zitko et al. (1977)
Coho salmon (Oncorhynchus kisutch)		96-h LC_{50}	22.2	(+),(+)-t	static	12			Mauck et al. (1976)
		96-h LC_{50}	9.4	(+),(+)-t	flow-through	12			Mauck et al. (1976)
Killifish (Oryzias latipes)	adult	48-h LC_{50}	87	technical	static	25			Miyamoto (1976)
	adult	48-h LC_{50}	50	(+)-trans	static	25			Miyamoto (1976)
	adult	48-h LC_{50}	42	(+)-cis	static	25			Miyamoto (1976)
	adult	48-h LC_{50}	32	(+),(+)-t	static	25			Miyamoto (1976)
Rainbow trout (Salmo gairdneri)		24-h LC_{50}	20	technical	static				Cope (1965)
		48-h LC_{50}	19	technical	static				Anon. (1968)
Steelhead trout (Salmo gairdneri)		96-h LC_{50}	17.5	(+),(+)-t	static	12			Mauck et al. (1976)
		96-h LC_{50}	9.70	(+),(+)-t	flow-through	12			Mauck et al. (1976)
Channel catfish (Ictalurus panctatus)		96-h LC_{50}	30.1	(+),(+)-t	static	12			Mauck et al. (1976)
		96-h LC_{50}	27.0	(+),(+)-t	flow-through	12			Mauck et al. (1976)
		96-h LC_{50}	14.6	(+),(+)-t	flow-through	12			Mauck et al. (1976)

Table 4 (contd).

Species	Size	Parameter	Concentration (µg/litre)	Formulation[a]	System	Temperature (°C)	pH	Hardness (mg $CaCO_3$/litre) or salinity (‰)	Reference
Fish (contd).									
Yellow perch (*Perca flavescens*)		96-h LC_{50}	9.90	(+), (+)-t	flow-through	12			Mauck et al. (1976)
		96-h LC_{50}	7.80	(+), (+)-t	static	12			Mauck et al. (1976)
Fathead minnow (*Pimephales promelas*)		96-h LC_{50}	80.0	(+), (+)-t	static	12			Mauck et al. (1976)
		96-h LC_{50}	53.0	(+), (+)-t	flow-through	12			Mauck et al. (1976)
Bluegill (*Lepomis macrochirus*)	0.8 g	96-h LC_{50}	35	(+), (+)-t	static	22	7.5	40 - 80	Mauck et al. (1976)
	0.8 g	96-h LC_{50}	47	(+), (+)-t	static	17	7.5	40 - 48	Mauck et al. (1976)
	0.8 g	96-h LC_{50}	56	(+), (+)-t	static	12	7.5	40 - 48	Mauck et al. (1976)
	0.8 g	96-h LC_{50}	49	(+), (+)-t	static	12	6.6	10 - 13	Mauck et al. (1976)
	0.8 g	96-h LC_{50}	49	(+), (+)-t	static	12	7.8	160 - 180	Mauck et al. (1976)
	0.8 g	96-h LC_{50}	42.5	(+), (+)-t	static	12	8.2	280 - 320	Mauck et al. (1976)
	0.8 g	96-h LC_{50}	56	(+), (+)-t	static	12	6.5	40 - 48	Mauck et al. (1976)
	0.8 g	96-h LC_{50}	60	(+), (+)-t	static	12	9.5	40 - 48	Mauck et al. (1976)
	0.8 g	96-h LC_{50}	27.6	(+), (+)-t	static	17	7.5	40 - 48	Mauck et al. (1976)
	0.8 g	96-h LC_{50}	33.2	(+), (+)-t	static	12	7.5	40 - 48	Mauck et al. (1976)

Table 4 (contd).

Fish (contd).									
Bluegill (*Lepomis macrochirus*) (contd)	0.8 g	96-h LC_{50}	39	(+), (+)-t	static	12	6.6	10 - 13	Mauck et al. (1976)
	0.8 g	96-h LC_{50}	30	(+), (+)-t	static	12	7.8	160 - 180	Mauck et al. (1976)
	0.8 g	96-h LC_{50}	36	(+), (+)-t	static	12	8.2	280 - 320	Mauck et al. (1976)
	0.8 g	96-h LC_{50}	25	(+), (+)-t	static	12	6.6	40 - 48	Mauck et al. (1976)
	0.8 g	96-h LC_{50}	25	(+), (+)-t	static	12	9.5	40 - 48	Mauck et al. (1976)
Arthropods									
Sigara substriata	0.59 cm; 6.1 mg	48-h LC_{50}	150	technical	static	25			Nishiuchi (1981)
Micronecta sedula	0.32 cm; 1.8 mg	48-h LC_{50}	420	technical	static	25			Nishiuchi (1981)
Cloeon dipterum	0.93 cm; 5.6 mg	48-h LC_{50}	350	technical	static	25			Nishiuchi (1981)
Orthetrum albistylum speciosum	2.3 cm; 0.62 g	48-h LC_{50}	1500	technical	static	25			Nishiuchi (1981)
Eretes sticticus	1.5 cm; 0.2 g	48-h LC_{50}	380	technical	static	25			Nishiuchi (1981)
Sympetrum frequens	2.1 cm; 0.56 g	48-h LC_{50}	1300	technical	static	25			Nishiuchi (1981)
	2.1 cm; 0.56 g	48-h LC_{50}	2000	technical	static	15			Nishiuchi (1981)
	2.1 cm; 0.56 g	48-h LC_{50}	2000	technical	static	20			Nishiuchi (1981)

Table 4 (contd).

Species	Size	Parameter	Concentration (µg/litre)	Formulation[a]	System	Temperature (°C)	pH	Hardness (mg $CaCO_3$/litre) or salinity (%)	Reference
Arthropods (contd).									
Sympetrum frequens (contd)	2.1 cm; 0.56 g	48-h LC_{50}	850	technical	static	30			Nishiuchi (1981)
Daphnia pulex		3-h LC_{50}	> 50 000	technical	static	25			Miyamoto (1976)
		3-h LC_{50}	> 50 000	(+)-cis	static	25			Miyamoto (1976)
		3-h LC_{50}	25 000 - 50 000	(+)-trans	static	25			Miyamoto (1976)
		3-h LC_{50}	5 000 - 10 000	(+).(+)-t	static	25			Miyamoto (1976)
		48-h EC_{50}	21						Sanders & Cope (1966)
Stonefly (Pteronarcys californica)		48-h LC_{50}	28	technical					Anon. (1968)
	3-3.5 cm	96-h LC_{50}	2.1	technical	static	15.5	7.1		Sanders & Cope (1968)
Gammarus lacustris		48-h LC_{50}	20						Anon. (1968)
		24-h LC_{50}	38						Sanders (1969)
Simocephalus serrulatus		48-h EC_{50}	56						Sanders & Cope (1966)

[a] (+).(+)-t = (+)-allethronyl (+)-trans allethrin = S-Bioallethrin.
(+)-trans = (+)-trans-allethrin = bioallethrin.
(+)-cis = (+)-cis-allethrin.

Table 5. Acute toxicity of allethrin for non-target terrestrial organisms

Species	Size	Application	Toxicity	Temperature (°C)	Reference
Birds					
Mallard (Anas platyrhynchos)	young	oral (in capsule)	LD_{50} > 2000 (mg/kg)		Tucker & Crabtree (1970)
Arthropods					
Honey-bee (Apis mellifera)		contact	LD_{50} 3.4 (μg/bee)	26 - 27	Stevenson et al. (1978)
		oral	LD_{50} 4.6-9.1 (μg/bee)		Stevenson et al. (1978)

6. EFFECTS ON EXPERIMENTAL ANIMALS AND IN VITRO TEST SYSTEMS

6.1 Acute Toxicity

The acute oral toxicity of allethrin isomers for rats is moderate to weak (378-2430 mg/kg) (Table 6). However, allethrin injected intravenously in rats or intracerebrally in mice caused severe poisoning syndrome with tremors.

Table 6. Acute oral toxicity of allethrin isomers

Compound	Animal	Sex	LD_{50} (mg/kg body weight)	Reference
Allethrin	rat	M	2430	Miyamoto (1976)
	rat	F	720	Miyamoto (1976)
	rat	M	920	Carpenter et al. (1950)
	rat	F	900	Carpenter et al. (1950)
	mouse	M	500	Miyamoto (1976)
	mouse	F	630	Miyamoto (1976)
	mouse	M	480[a]	Carpenter et al. (1950)
	mouse	F	1580[b]	Carpenter et al. (1950)
	rabbit	M	4290	Carpenter et al. (1950)
Bioallethrin	mouse	M	330	Miyamoto (1976)
	mouse	F	350	Miyamoto (1976)
	rat	M	709	Audegond et al. (1979a)
	rat	F	1041	Audegond et al. (1979a)
S-Bioallethrin	rat	M	1290	Miyamoto (1976)
	rat	F	430	Miyamoto (1976)
	rat	M	574	Audegond et al. (1979c)
	rat	F	412	Audegond et al. (1979c)
	mouse	M	285	Miyamoto (1976)
	mouse	F	250	Miyamoto (1976)
d-cis-Allethrin	mouse	M	210	Miyamoto (1976)
	mouse	F	270	Miyamoto (1976)
Esbiothrin	rat	M	432	Audegond et al. (1979b)
	rat	F	378	Audegond et al. (1979b)

[a] 20% in deodorized kerosene.
[b] 5% in deodorized kerosene.

When allethrin was applied to shaved skin on the backs of Wistar rats (8 females and 6 males/group) or ddY mice (10 females and 10 males/group) at dose levels of 2 g/kg body weight or 5 g/kg body weight, 8 out of 16 mice treated with 5 g/kg died, but none of the rats (Nakanishi et al., 1970).

Esbiothrin was applied to the shaved skin of New Zealand white male and female rabbits at a level of 2000 mg/kg body weight. All the animals showed erythema and, in some cases, an oedematous reaction, but behaviour and body weight gain remained normal. There were no compound-related deaths (Kaysen & Sales, 1984).

The minimum toxic doses of d-allethrin (2-h exposure) and S-Bioallethrin (3-h exposure) for rats and mice, exposed to each compound in the form of a mist, were: d-allethrin, rats - 260 mg/m^3, mice - 260 mg/m^3, S-Bioallethrin, rats - 24 mg/m^3, and mice - 91 mg/m^3 (Miyamoto, 1976).

Wistar male rats were exposed to atmospheres containing bioallethrin at 500, 1000, or 2000 mg/m^3 for 24 h. No deaths occurred throughout the trial. The no-observed-adverse-effect level via inhalation was 1000 mg/m^3, which is about 3000 times higher than the expected concentration under normal conditions of use (Chesher & Malone, 1972a).

Wistar male and female rats were exposed to respirable droplets of esbiothrin for a period of 4 h. There was no treatment-related change in the number of survivors, but congestion of the lungs was found in dead animals. The LC_{50} was 2630 mg/m^3 (Hardy et al., 1984).

Male and female ICR-JCL mice and Sprague Dawley rats were exposed to S-Bioallethrin in deotomisol via the inhalation route for 2 h. The LC_{50} was approximately 1500 mg/m^3 for mice and more than 1650 mg/m^3 for rats (Sakamoto et al., 1975c).

The acute inhalation toxicity (8 h/day for 3 consecutive days) of the smoke from S-Bioallethrin mosquite coils was extremely low for ICR mice and Sprague Dawley rats (Ogami et al., 1975). A smoke concentration 60 times that normally found did not induce toxic symptoms or death in either the mouse or the rat.

6.2 Short-term Studies

6.2.1 Allethrin

Rats showed a slight decrease in growth rate when fed commercial allethrin at a dietary level of 5000 mg/kg, while growth rate was nearly normal when the same concentration of purified allethrin was administered. It appeared that a dietary level of 2500 mg/kg did not produce any clinical effects. Examination of the liver was not reported (Ambrose & Robbins, 1951). Rats fed allethrin for 16 weeks did not show any gross effects at 5000 mg/kg, but showed tremors and convulsions at 10 000 mg/kg (Lehman, 1952).

When allethrin was given to Wistar rats at dietary levels of 1000, 5000, and 15 000 mg/kg for 12 weeks, a decrease in body-weight gain, an increase in liver or kidney weight ratio, and bile ductule proliferation were seen at levels of 5000 mg/kg or more. Similar observations were seen when 5000 mg

S-Bioallethrin/kg was administered to Sprague-Dawley rats for 12 weeks (Miyamoto, 1976).

Allethrin was administered via gastric intubation to male rats (10 animals in each group) at dose levels of 0, 250, 500, or 1000 mg/kg body weight per day, for 6 days a week over 12 weeks. At 1000 mg/kg, half the rats died following the first dose. No abnormal signs were observed in the remaining dosage groups. Higher relative weights of liver, thyroid (at 250 and 500 mg/kg), and kidney (at 500 mg/kg) were observed. Histopathological examination revealed papillary changes in the epithelium and hypertrophy of epithelial cells in the thyroids of rats at both 250 and 500 mg/kg (Nakanishi et al., 1970).

Four male and four female dogs fed allethrin at a rate of 50 mg/kg per day over 2 years did not show any gross or microscopic effects. Animals in other groups receiving higher doses suffered convulsions, survival time was progressively shortened, and non-specific pathological changes were observed (Lehman, 1965).

Rats (and dogs) withstood repeated inhalation of allethrin aerosols in air at a concentration several times higher than levels normally used. However, because of the method of administration, it was not possible to measure intake as mg/kg body weight (Carpenter et al., 1950).

Eight female mice inhaled allethrin at a level of 3 g/m^3 for 4 h/ day, 6 days a week, over 4 weeks. No deaths were observed. Eye discharge was seen in all animals after each exposure throughout the 4-week period. A slight, sporadic decrease in activity was found from the third week. Histopathological examination of the lungs of 5 mice showed bronchopneumonia (Nakanishi et al., 1970).

6.2.2 d-Allethrin

A 90-day toxicity study was conducted on Wistar rats (male and female) fed diets containing d-allethrin at 0, 750, 2000, or 4000 mg/kg. Increased liver weight was observed in animals receiving 2000 mg/kg or more and glutamine-oxaloacetic- and glutamine-pyruvic acid transaminase activities were raised in those receiving 4000 mg/kg.

The no-observed-adverse-effect dietary level for d-allethrin was 750 mg/kg diet (49.6 mg/kg body weight per day for male mice and 59.2 mg/kg per day for females) (Kadota, T., 1972).

ICR mice and Sprague-Dawley rats (both male and female) were exposed to a mist (particle diameter 1-2 µm, generated by means of atomizer) of d-allethrin (123 mg/m^3) or S-Bioallethrin (6.1, 16.9, or 61.3 mg/m^3) for 3 h per day, 5 days per week, over 4 weeks (Miyamoto, 1976). Mortality rates, behaviour, body and organ weights, haematology, clinical biochemistry, and histopathology of the organs were examined. Toxic symptoms, such as salivation and tremors, were found only in groups administered d-allethrin at 123 mg/m³ and S-Bioallethrin at 61.3 mg/m³.

In a study by Kadota et al. (1974), ICR mice and Sprague-Dawley rats were exposed to the smoke of mosquito coils containing 0.3% d-allethrin, at 20 times the conventional rate of application (10 coils/24 m³), in a closed room for 8 h/day, 6 days/week over 5 weeks. There were no effects on body and organ weights, food consumption, haematology, blood biochemistry, or histopathology.

6.2.3 Bioallethrin

Bioallethrin was given to groups of Wistar rats (16 males and 16 females) for 90 consecutive days at concentrations of 500, 1500, 5000, or 10 000 mg/kg diet (Wallwork et al., 1972). No marked adverse effects were observed, except for a slight to moderate decrease in body weight gain and slight liver dysfunction, observed in the groups receiving 5000 and 10 000 mg/kg, respectively. No dose-related macroscopic or microscopic changes were observed. The no-observed-adverse-effect level for bioallethrin in rats, after 90 days of treatment, was 1500 mg/kg diet (equivalent to an intake of about 135 mg/kg body weight per day).

Dogs were administered bioallethrin in the diet at concentrations of 200, 1000, or 5000 mg/kg for 6 months (Griggs et al., 1982). No animals died during the study. General body trembling and irregular heart rhythm were noted at the highest dose level. Body-weight gain was slightly reduced in males receiving 1000 mg/kg diet and in both sexes receiving 5000 mg/kg. Consistent elevation in the mean levels of alkaline phosphatase was noted at 1000 and 5000 mg/kg in males, at 5000 mg/kg in females, and an elevated SGPT at 5000 mg/kg was observed in both males and females. No compound-related macroscopic changes were observed. Histological investigation revealed hepatocellular degeneration in both males and females in the groups receiving 1000 and 5000 mg/kg. This was associated with intracanalicular and hepatocellular pigmentation. Similar pigmentation was seen within the tubular epithelium of the renal cortex. The no-observed-adverse-effect level in this study was 200 mg/kg diet (equivalent to an intake of 6.1 and 7.2 mg/kg (1.6 ml) per day for males and females, respectively).

No marked drug-related changes were observed in Wistar male rats exposed through continuous inhalation to a concentration of 125 mg bioallethrin/m³ air, for 10 consecutive days (Chesher & Malone, 1972b).

6.2.4 S-Bioallethrin

Groups of 10 Wistar rats (5 males and 5 females) were given S-Bioallethrin in the diet for 90 days; groups of 20 animals (10 males and 10 females) received S-Bioallethrin for 180 days (Motoyama et al., 1975a). Males received S-Bioallethrin at dietary levels of 3, 1, 0.3, or 0.1 g/kg, and females, at 1.5, 0.3, 0.1, or 0.05 g/kg. The differences in the doses between the sexes were due to the results of an acute toxicity study in which the LD_{50} for males was about 300 mg/kg and that for females, about 170 mg/kg. Abnormal symptoms were not observed, and deaths did not occur in either study. No macroscopic abnormal changes were observed. Histological investigation did not show any compound-related lesions, only scattered changes, which also occurred in the untreated groups and did not show any regular tendency. S-Bioallethrin did not induce any toxic effects in the males receiving the highest dose (3 g/kg) or in the females receiving the highest dose of 1.5 g/kg. The calculated doses of S-Bioallethrin for the males were about 330 mg/kg body weight in the early stages of the study and 200 mg/kg body weight in the later stages; the females received about 120 and 100 mg/kg body weight.

JLC-ICR mice and Sprague-Dawley rats were exposed for 2 h/day, 6 days a week, for a month to concentrations of S-Bioallethrin in deotomisol of 20 mg/m^3, 80 mg/m^3, or 160 mg/m^3. The lowest concentration was well tolerated. At 80 mg/m^3 and 160 mg/m^3, toxic signs, such as excitation, tail raising, jumping, salivation, and slight trembling occurred in the mice and slight salivation and nasal haemorrhage, in the rats. No changes were observed in haematological and biochemical tests or microscopically. S-Bioallethrin seemed to be more toxic in the mouse (1 death/24 at 80 mg/m^3 and 4 deaths/24 at 160 mg/m^3) than in the rat (no deaths) (Sakamoto et al., 1975d).

In a further study by Sakamoto et al. (1975b), JCL-ICR mice and JCL Sprague-Dawley rats were exposed for 8 h/day, 6 days a week, for 5 weeks to the smoke containing S-Bioallethrin emitted from 5 or 10 mosquito coils per 9.9 m^2 room area. The atmospheric concentrations produced were more than 10 or 20 times greater than would be found under normal conditions of use. Toxic effects were not observed in either the mouse or the rat and there were no deaths. The results indicate that the short-term inhalation toxicity of the fumes from S-Bioallethrin mosquito coils is extremely low (Sakamoto et al., 1975b).

Two studies with an S-Bioallethrin electric mosquito mat were performed on mice. Animals were exposed for 8 h per day, 6 days a week over 4 weeks, to fumes that were 25 or 10 times the concentration normally used. As treated animals in the first study showed encephalitis, a second study was performed to check whether the pathological changes were a specific effect of the product or a viral infection. Encephalitis did not occur in any of the treated animals (160 animals treated instead of 40) in the second study. Slight circulatory disorders in the brain and lungs and slight inflammation of the lungs were observed only in animals exposed to 25 times the normal concentration. The possibility that encephalitis was a specific effect of S-Bioallethrin was therefore dismissed (Tsuchiyama et al., 1975).

6.3 Primary Irritation

6.3.1 Eye irritation

Two solutions of allethrin dissolved in olive oil (10% and 50%) were prepared. One tenth ml of solution was applied to one eye of each test rabbit. Both dosages of allethrin produced eyelid-closure, slight conjunctival hyperaemia at 10 and 30 min, respectively, after application, and eye discharge 2 h after application. Lachrymation was also observed in the group treated with the 50% solution from 0.5 to 2 h after application (Nakanishi et al., 1970).

The effects of 0.1 ml undiluted esbiothrin were evaluated in 9 male albino New Zealand rabbits using the Draize test method and classified according to irritation potential by the Kay and Calandra scale, as modified by Guillot (Audegond et al., 1984b). The compound was classified as slightly irritant in both rinsed and unrinsed eyes.

When 0.1 ml undiluted S-Bioallethrin and 0.1 ml 50% solution of S-Bioallethrin in corn oil were applied to the eyes of male Japanese white rabbits, only slight eye irritation occurred (Sakamoto et al., 1975a). Symptoms included nictitation, hyperaemia of the conjunctiva, and tears. No abnormalities of the iris or cornea were observed.

6.3.2 Skin irritation

Undiluted technical allethrin (0.5 ml) or a 20% solution in olive oil (2.5 ml) were applied to the dorsal skin of rabbits. No differences were observed between allethrin-treated rabbits and the untreated controls (Nakanishi et al., 1970).

The dermal irritancy of a mixture of 4% bioallethrin and 20% piperonyl butoxide in an odourless petroleum distillate was evaluated on the intact and abraded skin of 3 California female rabbits, using the Draise test method. Virtually no reaction was produced on the intact skin, but increases in the degree of erythema and the duration of reaction were observed on the abraded skin. However, by 6 days, all treated sites were normal. Thus, bioallethrin was classified as mildly irritating on abraded skin (Vercoe & Malone, 1969).

In a similar study, the dermal irritancies of bioallethrin and of esbiothrin were determined on the intact and abraded skin of the rabbit, according to the Draize method (Motoyama et al., 1975b). Both compounds were found to be slightly irritant.

The primary dermal irritancy of a 5 ml dose of esbiothrin was evaluated over a 7-day test period on the intact and abraded skin of 6 male, albino New Zealand rabbits using the Draise test method. An increase in the degree of erythema was observed in both the intact and abraded skin, but by 7 days all treated sites were normal. Thus, esbiothrin was classified as slightly irritant (Audegond et al., 1984a).

In a study by Motoyama et al. (1975b), the primary dermal irritancy of S-Bioallethrin was evaluated for 72 h on the intact skin of 5 male and 5 female Wistar rats and 3 groups of 3 male and 3 female Nagano white rabbits. The doses administered to the rats included undiluted S-Bioallethrin and dilutions of 5 or 25 times in corn oil. The doses administered to the rabbits included undiluted S-Bioallethrin and dilutions of 10 or 100 times in corn oil. No changes were observed in the dermis of either the rat or the rabbit, at any dose level.

S-Bioallethrin produced mild primary irritation of the intact skin and the skin surrounding an abrasion in New Zealand white rabbits (details of the study not given in the report) (Fisch, 1974).

6.4 Sensitization

One half ml of a 5% olive oil solution of allethrin was applied topically to the backs of male guinea-pigs, every other day, 10 times. Two weeks after the last application, the animals were challenged with a similar application of allethrin. Only a sporadic pinkish colour was observed (same degree as vehicle control) at the site of application. Histopathological examination revealed slight lymphocytic and monocytic infiltration of the dermis in the allethrin-treated group (Nakanishi et al., 1970).

The sensitizing properties of a 10% solution of bioallethrin in petroleum distillate were evaluated in the Stevens ear-flank test in 2 groups of 10 male albino guinea-pigs (Saunders & Vercoe, 1970). Bioallethrin did not produce any irritation, but produced slight sensitization.

6.5 Long-term Studies and Carcinogenicity

When Wistar rats were exposed to racemic allethrin (dietary levels of 500, 1000, or 2000 mg/kg) for 80 weeks, bile duct proliferation was seen at levels of 1000 mg/kg or more and a decrease in glutamine-oxaloacetic acid transaminase activity was seen at 2000 mg/kg. However, no oncogenic effects were observed at any dose level (Miyamoto, 1976).

F344 rats (male and female) were fed diets containing d-allethrin at 0, 125, 500, or 2000 mg/kg for 123 weeks. Reduced body weight and increased liver and kidney weights were observed at levels exceeding 500 mg/kg and the activities of glutamine-oxaloacetic- and glutamine-pyruvic acid transaminase and alkaline phosphatase decreased at these levels. Histopathological examination showed histiocytes phagocyting crystals in the liver of animals fed levels of 500 mg/kg or more, but no oncogenic effects were observed at any dose level. The no-observed-adverse-effect level was 125 mg/kg, i.e., 5.9 mg/kg body weight per day (male) and 6.6 mg/kg per day (female) (Sato et al., 1985).

6.6 Mutagenicity and Related End-points

The mutagenic potential of allethrin has been examined in a wide range of tests including *in vitro/in vivo* gene mutation, DNA damage and repair, and *in vitro/in vivo* structural chromosomal aberration (Suzuki, 1975; Miyamoto, 1976; Suzuki, 1979; Kawachi et al., 1979; Kishida & Suzuki, 1979; Matsuoka et al., 1979; Hara & Suzuki, 1980; Sasaki et al., 1980; Kimmel et al., 1982; Garret et al., 1986). The results of all tests were negative with the exception of a gene mutation *Salmonella typhimurium* study with metabolic activation and a chromosomal aberration study on Chinese hamster cells (Matsuoka, et al., 1979; Kimmel et al., 1982). Both studies are considered inadequate because, in the gene mutation study the results were found to be attributable to photoproducts in improperly stored samples and, in the second study, the purity of the test material was not identified (Isobe et al., 1982, 1984).

Bioallethrin and esbiothrin were also tested for mutagenicity in both *in vitro* mammalian test systems, the micronucleus test system, and microbial assays and found to be negative (Peyre et al., 1979; Chantot & Vannier, 1984; Richold et al., 1984; Vannier & Fournex, 1984).

6.7 Reproductive Effects, Embryotoxicity, and Teratogenicity

When allethrins were administered to ICR mice during gestation to examine maternal and embryotoxic effects (Table 7),

Table 7. Teratological studies on allethrins isomers

Compound	Animals[a]	Dose mg/kg body weight per day	Route	Administration (days of gestation)
d-Allethrin	mouse	15,50,150	oral	7-12
S-Bioallethrin	mouse	10,30,100	oral	7-12

[a] Includes breeding of naturally delivered offspring.

no significant adverse effects, such as abortion or resorption of the fetus or embryo, external or skeletal abnormalities of pups, or abnormalities in growth and organ differentiation, were observed at the doses tested (Miyamoto, 1976).

Allethrin in corn oil was administered daily, by oral intubation, to pregnant albino rabbits from day 6 to day 18 of gestation at levels of 0 mg/kg (controls - corn oil only), 215 mg/kg (low level), and 350 mg/kg (high level). There were no indications of compound related effects among the test animals, which were similar to the controls in appearance, behaviour, body weight gain, and food consumption; necropsy findings were also similar.

The number of implantation sites compared with the number of ovarian corpora lutea observed was similar in the pregnant animals in control, low-dose, and high-dose groups. The number and placement of implantation sites, the resorption sites, the numbers of live and dead fetuses, and the fetal weights and lengths were also similar in the control and test animals. Fetal skeletal evaluations did not reveal any compound-related abnormalities or trends towards lesser or greater development in the test fetuses compared with the controls. Pups, of low- and high-dose animals, delivered naturally, were similar in appearance, external morphology, and behaviour. No compound-related observations were found during the post-delivery period (40 days) or at necropsy of the pups (Weatherholtz, 1972).

Bioallethrin was administered orally to pregnant Sprague-Dawley rats from day 6 to day 15 of gestation at levels of 50, 125, or 195 mg/kg body weight per day (Knickerbocker & Thomas, 1979). At 195 mg/kg, maternal mortality was increased, but there were no effects on dam body weight or weight gain during gestation. The compound did not have any effects on pregnancy, implantations, number of live fetuses, number of dead fetuses, or number of resorption sites per dam. Skeletal examination of fetuses revealed a significant increase in the number of litters with rudimentary 14 ribs at 50, 125, and 195 mg/kg as well as missing sternebrae at 50 mg/kg. However, these abnormalities were generally variations rather than malformations. No soft-tissue abnormalities were ascribed to treatment.

S-Bioallethrin was administered to pregnant Wistar rats from day 9 to day 14 of gestation at the following doses: 0.025, 0.05, 0.1, or 0.2 ml/kg body weight (Shinoda et al., 1975). The mortality rate at the dose of 0.2 ml/kg was 55%; at 0.01 and 0.05 ml/kg, the mortality rates were 4 and 5%, respectively. There were no differences between the control and treated groups in the numbers of implantations and live fetuses, and the frequency of fetal death. The weights of live fetuses and the placenta from the group administered 0.2 ml/kg were lower than those of the control group. Fetal and placental weights in the groups receiving 0.1, 0.05, or 0.025 ml/kg were almost the same as those in the control group. External abnormalities consisted of a cleft palate in one fetus and a decreased number of digits in 7 fetuses from the same pregnant dam (0.2 ml/kg). Skeletal abnormalities included lumbar transforming into thoracic vertebrae and insufficient ossification of the 5th sternebra; they were frequently observed in all groups but appeared to be dose-related. Some other abnormalities observed in a small number of fetuses from the treated groups included partial fusion of the cervical vertebrae or of vertebrae arches and ribs in the same fetuses in the 0.2 ml/kg group. Because of their low frequency, these abnormalities could not be attributed to treatment. In conclusion, S-Bioallethrin did not seem to induce any disorders in the fetuses of pregnant rats administered doses equal to or lower than 0.1 ml/kg, although some variations were observed at the 0.2 mg/kg level.

Shinoda et al. (1975) also administered S-Bioallethrin orally at 0.05, 0.1, or 0.2 ml/kg to pregnant TVCS mice from day 7 to day 12 of gestation. The mortality rate at 0.2 ml/kg was 40% and pregnancy was maintained in only one dam. Some toxic symptoms were observed at 0.1 ml/kg, and the mortality rate was 7%. The numbers of implantations and of viable fetuses, the sex ratio, placental and fetal weights in groups treated with 0.1 or 0.05 ml/kg, did not differ from those of the control group. External examination revealed that 2 fetuses from the 0.1 ml/kg treated group had cleft palates; one of them had hydrocephaly. These abnormalities could not be attributed to treatment because of their very low incidence and the presence in the control group of one fetus with an abdominal hernia and one with a cleft palate. There were not any skeletal abnormalities that could be related to treatment. In conclusion, at the maximum tolerated doses of

S-Bioallethrin of 0.1 ml/kg and 0.05 ml/kg, no lethal effects occurred in the embryos or fetuses and no teratogenic effects were observed.

6.8 Potentiation

Potentiation of toxicity between bioallethrin and piperonyl butoxide was studied by the intraperitoneal route in the rat (Wallwork & Malone, 1969). The degree of potentiation between the 2 compounds was very low.

6.9 Mechanism of Toxicity - Mode of Action

The toxic effects of allethrin result from its action on the nervous system. After intravenous injection with a lethal dose of bioallethrin (4 mg/kg body weight), initial tremors were followed by death within 20 min. Hyperexcitation and tremors usually developed a few minutes after application (Verschoyle & Barnes, 1972; Carlton, 1977; Wouters & Van den Bercken, 1978; Verschoyle & Aldridge, 1980; Lawrence & Casida, 1982). Signs of poisoning in vertebrates, including mammals, are similar to those in insects (see Appendix).

Signs of poisoning in insects generally include hyperexcitation, tremors, and convulsions, followed later by paralysis and death. Narahashi (1969, 1971) examined signs of poisoning electrophysiologically using the giant axon of the cockroach. Allethrin caused an increase in negative afterpotential, repetitive discharge (or repetitive firing) following electrical stimulation, and a conduction block, presumably by allethrin binding to sodium channels. Good correlations existed in cockroaches between the signs induced by allethrin and effects on the nervous system. Restless behaviour, without a loss of coordination, was correlated with repetitive discharge of cercal sensory neurons, whereas the onset of uncoordinated behaviour coincided with the appearance of abnormal discharges, not only in cercal sensory neurons but also in motor neurons and the central nervous system (CNS) (Gammon, 1979). Temperature had a profound effect on allethrin-induced repetitive discharges and its nerve-blocking action. In the giant axon of the cockroach treated with allethrin, repetitive discharges appeared at over 26.5 °C and increased with rise in temperature. Conversely, allethrin blocked the action potential of the squid and cockroach giant axons more strongly at 8 °C than at 23 °C (Wang et al., 1972). The negative temperature coefficient of the nerve-blocking action of allethrin appears to be responsible for a greater killing effect on insects, and is in sharp contrast with the positive temperature coefficient of repetitive discharges, which may be responsible for knock-down (Wang et al., 1972; Starkus & Narahashi, 1978). When the temperature was reduced from 23 to 8 °C in the voltage clamp analysis, the inhibition of the transient sodium conductance and the shift of the sodium conductance curve along the potential axis in the direction of hyperpolarization were both increased, causing a greater blocking of action potential (Narahashi, 1976).

However, it has been reported that the peripheral nerves of the rat and the frog were fairly insensitive to the blocking action of allethrin, and it was tentatively suggested that the nerve membranes of vertebrates were less susceptible to the neurotoxic action of allethrin than those of invertebrates. Allethrin causes a depolarizing after-potential following the action potential and induces pronounced repetitive firing in myelinated nerve fibres and in the sense organs of frogs. In the frog peripheral nervous system, virtually no blocking effect of allethrin occurs, except at very high concentrations (Van den Bercken et al., 1979).

The sodium channel gating model was proposed by Van den Bercken & Vijverberg (1980). The state of the sodium channel is controlled by 2 independent gates called the activation gate (or m-gate) and the inactivation gate (or h-gate), both of which are dependent on the membrane potential, but in opposite ways. The action of allethrin has been thought to stabilize the m-gate in its open position.

Pyrethroids were classified into 2 classes based on the signs and symptoms produced by acutely-toxic doses in mammals (Verschoyle & Aldridge, 1980; Lawrence & Casida, 1982) and on the neurophysiological responses in cockroaches (Gammon et al., 1981). Type I syndrome involves hyperactivity and tremor in both insects and mammals. Type II syndrome involves hyperactivity, incoordination, and convulsions in insects, and clonic seizures with sinuous writhing (choreoathetosis) in mammals. Allethrin is classified as a Type I compound.

Interactions of allethrin with the nicotinic acetylcholine (ACh) receptor channel were studied in membranes from the Torpedo electric organ (Abbassy et al., 1982). Allethrin did not inhibit binding of [^{3}H]-ACh to the receptor sites, but noncompetitively inhibited binding of [^{3}H] perhydrohistrionico-toxin ([^{3}H]H_{12}-HTX) to the ionic channel sites in a dose-dependent manner. The inhibition constant (K_i) of [^{3}H]H_{12}-HTX binding in the absence of receptor agonists was 30 µmol/litre while, in the presence of 100 µmol carbamylcholine/litre, it was 4 µmol/litre. This inhibitory effect of allethrin had a negative temperature coefficient. The high affinity binding of allethrin to the channel sites of the nicotinic ACh-receptor may be indicative of a postsynaptic site of action for allethrin, in addition to the known action on the sodium channel.

The mechanism of interaction of the 2 pyrethroids, allethrin and fluvalinate, with the nicotinic acetylcholine (ACh) receptor was investigated by means of their effects on the binding of radioligands to the *Torpedo* electric organ receptor and tracer ion flux. The data suggest that allethrin and fluvalinate bind to sites on the nicotinic ACh-receptor that are quite distinct from the receptor site and the ionic channel sites where noncompetitive blockers (e.g., $[^3H]H_{12}HTX$) bind. Such pyrethroids may be binding to sites that normally bind Ca^{2+} and induce receptor desensitization. The data imply that modulation of the nicotinic ACh-receptor in insect ganglia may be involved in the mode of action of pyrethroids (Sherby et al., 1986).

7. EFFECTS ON MAN

No data were available to the Task Group on the effects of allethrins on man. However, allethrins have been used for many years and no toxic effects on human beings have been reported.

8. EVALUATION OF HUMAN HEALTH RISKS AND EFFECTS ON THE ENVIRONMENT

8.1 Evaluation of Human Health Risks

Allethrin, consisting of 8 stereo-isomers, is an effective insecticide mainly used to control household insects.

d-Allethrin, bioallethrin, esbiothrin, and S-Bioallethrin are also available as selected stereo-isomers or mixtures thereof. It is anticipated that human exposure will be mainly through the inhalation of mists from aerosol sprays and from other household uses, such as the electric mat and mosquito coil. The air level following conventional household aerosol spraying of allethrin is not expected to exceed 0.5 mg/m³. Air levels of individual isomers are expected to be lower under similar conditions of use.

Although the levels of allethrins in food have not been determined, on the basis of current use patterns, it is unlikely that such dietary exposure will be significant.

No data are available on occupational exposure to the allethrins. In fact, though they have been used for many years, no data have been reported on their toxicity for human beings. Thus, extrapolation of data from experimental animals and in vitro studies must be relied on.

The results of short-term studies on experimental animals suggest that allethrins are weakly to moderately toxic (oral or dermal LD_{50} values of 210 - 4290 mg/kg; inhalation LC_{50} value of > 1500 mg/m³).

Allethrins induce mild primary eye and skin irritation in rabbits, but no skin sensitization.

The short-term toxicities of S-Bioallethrin and d-allethrin appear to be low, according to several inhalation studies (mosquito coil and mat) on mice and rats at a range of dose levels (10, 20, or 25 times normal concentration used).

The allethrins are not mutagenic in a variety of test systems including gene mutations, DNA damage and repair, and chromosomal effects.

d-Allethrin was not carcinogenic for rats fed diets containing 2000 mg/kg over 2 years.

Relatively high doses of allethrin, bioallethrin, or S-Bioallethrin were neither embryotoxic nor teratogenic for rabbits, rats, or mice. No adequate reproduction studies have been reported.

At near lethal doses, allethrins are likely to cause hyperactivity, tremors, and convulsions and have been classified as Type I pyrethroids.

No-observed-adverse-effect levels were established for bioallethrin in a 90-day rat study and a 6-month study on dogs

(1500 mg/kg diet, 200 mg/kg diet, respectively, corresponding to 135 mg/kg body weight and 6.1-7.2 mg/kg body weight, respectively). In a 2-year study on rats, the no-observed-adverse-effect level for dietary administration of allethrin was 125 mg/kg, i.e., 5.9 and 6.6 mg/kg body weight per day for male and female rats, respectively.

8.2 Evaluation of Effects on the Environment

Allethrins are primarily used indoors, but no information is available on levels in the environment. They are rapidly decomposed when exposed to sunlight and at temperatures exceeding 400 °C, but vaporize with slow heating at 150 °C.

Allethrins are toxic for fish with LC_{50} values of 9-90 µg/litre, but less toxic for *Daphnia* and aquatic insect larvae (150-50 000 µg/litre). Toxicity is low for birds (LD_{50} > 2000 mg/kg), but high for honey-bees (LD_{50} 3-9 µg/bee).

9. CONCLUSIONS

General population: Under recommended conditions of use, the exposure of the general population to allethrins is negligible and is unlikely to present a hazard.

Occupational exposure: With reasonable work practices, hygiene measures, and safety precautions, the use of allethrins is unlikely to present a hazard to those occupationally exposed to them.

Environment: Under recommended conditions of use and application rates, it is unlikely that allethrins or their degradation products will attain significant levels in the environment. In spite of the high toxicity of these compounds for fish and honey-bees, they are only likely to cause a problem in the case of spillage or misuse.

10. RECOMMENDATIONS

- Over 25 years of use, no adverse effects have been reported to arise from human exposure to allethrins, but it is still necessary to continue observations on human exposure.

- To improve the overall assessment of the potential reproductive effects and potential carcinogenic effects of the allethrins, it is suggested that consideration should be given to conducting an appropriate multigeneration study and another carcinogenicity study on a second species.

- The label for the household use of allethrins should include adequate instructions for use and storage and, where appropriate, warning of flammability.

- Efforts should be made to obtain a more precise estimate of the total global usage of allethrins.

11. PREVIOUS EVALUATIONS BY INTERNATIONAL BODIES

The Joint FAO/WHO Meeting on Pesticide Residues (JMPR) discussed and evaluated allethrin in 1965 (FAO/WHO, 1965). It did not establish an ADI for allethrin, because data from long-term studies were not available.

The Pesticide Development and Safe Use Unit, Division of Vector Biology and Control, WHO, classified the acute hazard to health for technical allethrin as slight and for technical bioallethrin as moderate (WHO, 1986).

REFERENCES

ABBASSY, M.A., ELDENFRAWI, M.E., & ELDENFRAWI, T. (1982) Allethrin interactions with the nicotinic acetylcholine receptor channel. Life Sci., 31: 1547-1552.

AMBROSE, A.M. & ROBBINS, D.J. (1951) Comparative toxicity of pyrethrins and allethrin. Fed. Proc., 10: 276.

ANONYMOUS (1968) Official document of US Department of the Interior (USDI), Washington, DC, Federation of the Water Pollution Control Administration, US Department of the Interior, p. 234.

AUDEGOND, L., COLLAS, E., & GLOMOT, R. (1979a) Bioallethrin. Acute oral toxicity study in the rat, Romainville, France, Roussel Uclaf, 26 pp (Report No. RU-BA-79.829/A) (Unpublished proprietary data).

AUDEGOND, L., COLLAS, E., & GLOMOT, R. (1979b) Esbiothrin. Acute oral toxicity study in the rat, Romainville, France, Roussel Uclaf, 27 pp (Report No. RU-EBT-79.828/A) (Unpublished proprietary data).

AUDEGOND, L., COLLAS, E., & GLOMOT, R. (1979c) Esbiol. Acute oral toxicity study in the rat, Romainville, France, Roussel Uclaf, 30 pp (Report No. RU-SB-79.830/A) (Unpublished proprietary data).

AUDEGOND, L., COLLAS, E., & FOURNEX, R. (1984a) Esbiothrin. Primary dermal irritancy study in the male rabbit, Romainville, France, Roussel Uclaf, 12 pp (Report No. RU-EBT-83315/A) (Unpublished proprietary data).

AUDEGOND, L., COLLAS, E., & FOURNEX, R. (1984b) Esbiothrin. Primary eye irritation study in the male rabbit, Romainville, France, Roussel Uclaf, 16 pp (Report No. RU-EBT-83.316/A) (Unpublished proprietary data).

BABA, N. & OHNO, M. (1972) Thermal behavior of allethrin at 150 °C in atmospheric environment. Agric. biol. Chem., 36: 56-61.

BATTELLE (1982) Pesticide programme of research and market planning. Part I. Insecticides, Geneva, Battelle Institute (October 1982).

BULLIVALENT, M.J. & PATTENDEN, G. (1973) Photolysis of bioallethrin. Tetrahedron Lett., 38: 3679-3680.

CARLTON, M. (1977) Some effects of cismethrin on the rabbit nervous system. Pestic. Sci., 8: 700-712.

CARPENTER, C.P., WEIL, C.S., POZZANI, U.C., & SMYTH, J.F., Jr (1950) Comparative acute and subacute toxicities of allethrin and pyrethrins. Arch. ind. Hyg., 2: 420-432.

CHANTOT, J.F. & VANNIER, B. (1984) Esbiothrin. Detection of a mutagenic potency with a bacterial test (Ames test), Romainville, France, Roussel Uclaf, 14 pp (Report No. RU-EBT-84.04/A) (Unpublished proprietary data).

CHEN, Y.L. & CASIDA, J.E. (1969) Photodecomposition of pyrethrin I, allethrin, phthalthrin and dimethrin. Modification in the acid moiety. J. agric. food Chem., 17: 208-215.

CHESHER, B.C. & MALONE, J.C. (1972a) Bioallethrin. 24 hour exposure rat inhalation study, Berkhamsted, United Kingdom, Wellcome Foundation Ltd, 42 pp (Report No. WELL-BA-72.23.03/A) (Unpublished proprietary data supplied by Roussel Uclaf).

CHESHER, B.C. & MALONE, J.C. (1972b) Bioallethrin. 10 consecutive days rat inhalation, Berkhamsted, United Kingdom, Wellcome Foundation Ltd, 41 pp (Report No. WELL-BA-72.28.03/A) (Unpublished proprietary data supplied by Roussel Uclaf).

COPE, O.B. (1965) Sport fishery investigation, in the effects of pesticides on fish and wildlife. US Fish Wildl. Serv. Circ., 226: 51-64.

DESMARCHELIER, J.M. (1976) Analysis of pyrethroids on grains. J. stored Prod. Res., 12: 245-252.

DEVAUX, Ph. & BOLLA, P. (1986a) Bioallethrin. Water solubility, Romainville, France, Roussel Uclaf, 5 pp (Report No. STE-BA-057.07.1/A) (Unpublished proprietary data).

DEVAUX, Ph. & BOLLA, P. (1986b) Bioallethrin. n-octanol/water partition coefficient, Romainville, France, Roussel Uclaf, 4 pp (Report No. STE-BA-057.C.06.1/A) (Unpublished proprietary data).

DEVAUX, Ph. & TILLIER, C. (1986) Vapour pressure of bioallethrin and bioresmethrin, Romainville, France, Roussel Uclaf, 8 pp (Report No. RU-BRM/BA-150.06.86.STE/A) (Unpublished proprietary data).

ELLIOTT, M. (1977) Synthetic pyrethroids, Washington, DC, American Chemical Society, 229 pp (ACS Symposium Series No. 42).

ELLIOTT, M., JANES, N.F., CASIDA, J.E., & KIMMEL, E.C. (1972a) Mammalian metabolites of pyrethroids. Pyrethrum Post, 11: 94-103.

ELLIOTT, M., JANES, N.F., KIMMEL, E.C., & CASIDA, J.E. (1972b) Metabolic fate of pyrethrin I, pyrethrin II and allethrin administered orally to rats. J. agric. food Chem., 20: 300-313.

EVANS, M.H. (1976) End-plate potentials in frog muscle exposed to a synthetic pyrethroid. Pestic. Biochem. Physiol., 6: 547-550.

FAO (1982) Second Government Consultation on International Harmonization of Pesticide Registration Requirements, Rome, 11-15 October, 1982, Rome, Food and Agriculture Organization of the United Nations.

FAO/WHO (1965) Allethrin. In: Evaluation of the toxicity of pesticide residues in food, Rome, Food and Agriculture Organization of the United Nations, pp. 20-23 (FAO Meeting Report No. PL/1965/10/1 - WHO Food Add./27.65).

FISCH, H. (1974) Primary irritation evaluation program study, Springfield, National Technical Information Service, p. 4 (NTIS Report No. 51-029-75).

FLANNIGAN, S.A. & TUCKER, S.B. (1985) Variation in cutaneous sensation between synthetic pyrethroid insecticides. Contact Dermatitis, 13: 140-147.

GAMMON, D.W. (1979) An analysis of the temperature-dependence of the toxicity of allethrin to the cockroach. In: Narahashi, T., ed. Neurotoxicology of insecticides and pheromones, New York, Plenum Press, pp. 97-117.

GAMMON, D.W. & CASIDA, J.E. (1983) Pyrethroids of the most potent class antagonize GABA action at the crayfish neuromuscular junction. Neurosci. Lett., 40: 163-168.

GAMMON, D.W., BROWN, M.A., & CASIDA, J.E. (1981) Two classes of pyrethroid action in the cockroach. Pestic. Biochem. Physiol., 15: 181-191.

GAMMON, D.W., LAWRENCE, L.J., & CASIDA, J.E. (1982) Pyrethroids toxicology: Protective effects of Diazepam and phenobarbital in the mouse and the cockroach. Toxicol. appl. Pharmacol., 66: 290-296.

GARRET, N.E., FRANK STACK, H., & WATERS, M.D. (1986) Evaluation of the genetic activity profiles of 65 pesticides. Mutat. Res., 168: 301-325.

GLICKMAN, A.H. & CASIDA, J.E. (1982) Species and structural variations affecting pyrethroid neurotoxicity. Neurobehav. Toxicol. Teratol., 4: 793-799.

GRIGGS, M.P., JEFFERSON, N.D., BLAIR, M., & SPICER, E.J.F. (1982) Bioallethrin. 6-month dietary toxicity study in dogs, IRDC Mattawan, Michigan, 69 pp (Report No. IRDC-BA-406.034/A) (Unpublished proprietary data supplied by Roussel Uclaf).

HARA, M. & SUZUKI, H. (1980) In vivo chromosomal aberration test of allethrin on mouse bone marrow cells, Takarazuka, Sumitomo Chemical Co., Ltd (Report No. KT-00-0056) (Unpublished proprietary data).

HARDY, C.J., JACKSON, G.C., LEWIS, D.J., & GOPINATH, C. (1984) Esbiothrin (RU 27436). Acute inhalation toxicity in rats 4-hour exposure, Huntingdon, United Kingdom, Huntingdon Research Centre, 118 pp (Report No. RSL-EBT-84.470/A) (Unpublished proprietary data supplied by Roussel Uclaf).

ISOBE, N., MIHARA, K., SUZUKI, H., MATSUO, M., & MIYAMOTO, J. (1982) Identification of a mutagen in photooxidation products of allethrin, Takarazuka, Research Department, Pesticide Division, Sumitomo Chemical Co., Ltd (Technical Report No. 57-7-28) (Proprietary data made available by Sumitomo Chemical Co., Ltd).

ISOBE, N., MATSUO, M., & MIYAMOTO, J. (1984) Nevel photoproducts of allethrin. Tetrahedron Lett., 25: 861-864.

JAPAN PLANT PROTECTION ASSOCIATION (1984) [Pesticide manual] (Noyaku Yoran), Tokyo, Japan Plant Protection Association, p. 5 (in Japanese).

KADOTA, T. (1972) 90-day subacute toxicity study of Pynamin Forte on rats, Takarazuka, Research Department, Pesticide Division, Sumitomo Chemical Co., Ltd (Technical Report No. KT-70-0006) (Proprietary data made available by Sumitomo Chemical Co., Ltd).

KADOTA, T., KOHDA, H., & MIYAMOTO, J. (1974) Subacute inhalation toxicity study of mosquito coils containing 0.3% Pynamin Forte in mice and rats, Hyogo, Research Department, Pesticide Division, Sumitomo Chemical Co., Ltd (Technical Report No. KT-40-0031).

KAWACHI, T., YAHAGI, T., KADA, T., TAZIMA, Y., ISHIDATE, M., SASAKI, M., & SUGIYAMA, T. (1979) Cooperative programme on short-term assays for carcinogenicity in Japan. In: Montesano, R., Bartsch, H., & Tomatis, L., ed. Molecular and cellular aspects of carcinogen screening tests, Lyons, International Agency for Research on Cancer, pp. 323-330 (IARC Scientific Publications No. 27).

KAWANO, Y., YANAGIHARA, K., MIYAMOTO, T., & YAMAMOTO, I. (1980) Examination of the conversion products of pyrethrins and allethrin formulations exposed to sunlight by gas chromatography and mass spectroscopy. J. Chromatogr., 198: 317-328.

KAYSEN, A. & SALES, A. (1984) Esbiothrin. Acute dermal toxicity in male and female rabbits, Evreux, France, Centre International de Toxicologie, 36 pp (Report No. CIT-EBT-430.84/A) (Unpublished proprietary data supplied by Roussel Uclaf)

KIMMEL, E.C., CASIDA, J.E., & RUZO, L.O. (1982) Identification of mutagenic photoproducts of pyrethroids allethrin and terallethrin. J. agric. food Chem., 30: 623-626.

KISHIDA, F. & SUZUKI, H. (1979) Mutagenicity test of allethrin in bacterial test systems, Takarazuka, Research Department, Pesticide Division, Sumitomo Chemical Co., Ltd (Technical Report No. KT-90-0054) (Unpublished proprietary data made available by Sumitomo Chemical Co., Ltd).

KNICKERBOCKER, M. & THOMAS, A.R. (1979) Teratological evaluation of d-trans allethrin in Sprague-Dawley rats, USA, FDRL, 37 pp (Report No. FDRL-BA-79.20.04/A) (Unpublished proprietary data supplied by Roussel Uclaf).

KYOGOKU, K., IGUCHI, T., YAMAGUCHI, H., & MURAYAMA, H. (1970) Studies of pyrethroid insecticides. Part IV. Pyrolysis gas chromatography of allethrin, phthalthrin and other chrysanthemic acid esters. Nippon Nogeikagaku Kaishi, 44: 532-537.

LAWRENCE, L.J. & CASIDA, J.E. (1982) Pyrethroid toxicology: Mouse intracerebral structure-toxicity relationship. Pestic. Biochem. Physiol., 18: 9-14.

LAWRENCE, L.J. & CASIDA, J.E. (1983) Stereospecific action of pyrethroid insecticides on the gamma-aminobutyric acid receptor-ionophore complex. Science, 221: 1399-1401.

LAWRENCE, L.J., GEE, K.W., & YAMAMURA, H.I. (1985) Interactions of pyrethroid insecticides with chloride ionophore-associated binding sites. Neurotoxicology, 6: 87-98.

LEAHEY, J.P. (1985) The pyrethroid insecticides, London, Taylor & Francis, 440 pp.

LEHMAN, A.J. (1952) Summaries of pesticide toxicity, Q. Bull. Assoc. Food Drug Off., 16: 47.

LEHMAN, A.J. (1965) Summaries of pesticide toxicity, Topeca, Kansas, US Association of Food and Drug Officers.

LUND, A.E. & NARAHASHI, T. (1983) Kinetics of sodium channel modification as the basis for the variation in the serve membrane effects of pyrethroids and DDT analogs. Pestic. Biochem. Physiol., 20: 203-216.

MCCLELLAN, D.B. & MOORE, J.B. (1958) Determination of allethrin residues in milk and meats. J. agric. food Chem., 6: 463-465.

MARTIN, H. & WORTHING, C.R. (1977) The pesticide manual, 5th ed., Croydon, British Crop Protection Council, p. 7.

MATSUOKA, A., HAYASHI, M., & ISHIDATE, M. (1979) Chromosomal aberration test on 29 chemicals combined with S9 mix in vitro. Mutat. Res., 66: 277-290.

MAUCK, W.L., OLSON, L.E., & MARKING, L.L. (1976) Toxicity of natural pyrethroids and five pyrethroids to fish. Arch. environ. Contam. Toxicol., 4: 18-29.

MEISTER, R.T., BERG, G.L., SINE, C., MEISTER, S., & POPLYK, J. (1983) Farm chemicals handbook. Section C. Pesticide dictionary, Willoughby, Meister Publishing Co., pp. C10-C11.

MIYAMOTO, J. (1976) Degradation and metabolism and toxicity of synthetic pyrethroids. Environ. Health Perspect., 14: 15-28.

MIYAMOTO, J. (1981) The chemistry, metabolism and residue analysis of synthetic pyrethroids. Pure appl. Chem., 53: 1967-2022.

MIYAMOTO, J. & KEARNEY, P.C. (1983) Pesticide chemistry-human welfare and the environment. Proceedings of the Fifth International Congress of Pesticide Chemistry, Kyoto, Japan, 29 August-4 September, 1982, Oxford, Pergamon Press (in 4 volumes).

MOTOYAMA, I., YANAGIDAIRA, T., SAKAI, A., MINAKAMI, T., & TAGUCHI, H. (1975a) Esbiol. The results of subacute and chronic toxicity tests in the rat (6-month study), Shinshu, Japan, Shinshu University Medical College, 54 pp (Report No. SU-SB-75.07.19/A) (Unpublished proprietary data supplied by Roussel Uclaf).

MOTOYAMA, I., YANAGIDAIRA, T., SAKAI, A., & MINAKAMI, T. (1975b) Esbiol. Skin irritant tests in rabbits and rats, Shinshu, Japan, Shinshu University Medical College, 4 pp (Report No. SV-SB-75.07.24/A) (Unpublished proprietary data supplied by Roussel Uclaf).

MURANO, A. (1972) Determination of the optical isomers of insecticidal pyrethroids by gas-liquid chromatography. Agric. biol. Chem., 36: 2203-2211.

NAKADA, Y., YURA, Y., & MURAYAMA, K. (1971) Pyrolysis of allethrin. Bull. Chem. Soc. Jpn, 44: 1724.

NAKANISHI, M., MUKAI, T., TAKEUCHI, M., & EDANAGA, M. (1970) Toxicological studies on a new pyrethroid: Kikuthrin. Part I. Studies on insecticide V. Botyu-Kagaku, 35: 103-112.

NARAHASHI, T. (1969) Mode of action of DDT and allethrin on nerve: cellular and molecular mechanisms. Residue Rev., 25: 275-288.

NARAHASHI, T. (1971) Mode of action of pyrethroids. Bull. World Health Organ., 44: 337-345.

NARAHASHI, T. (1976) Nerve membrane as a target of pyrethroids. Pestic. Sci., 7: 267-272.

NIOSH (1983) In: Tatken, R.L. & Lewis, R.J., Jr, ed. Registry of toxic effects of chemical substances, 1981-82 edition, Cincinnati, Ohio, National Institute for Occupational Safety and Health, 3057 pp.

NISHIUCHI, Y. (1981) Toxicity of pesticides to some aquatic organisms. I. Toxicity of pesticides to some aquatic insects. Seitai-kagaku, 4: 31-46.

OGAMI, H., SHIMADA, T., & KAMITAMARI, M. (1975) Esbiol mosquito coils acute inhalation toxicity tests in the mouse and rat, Japan, Japan Mosquito Coil Co., Ltd, 9 pp (Report No. BRD-SB-75-02.25/A) (Unpublished proprietary data supplied by Roussel Uclaf).

PEYRE, M., CHANTOT, J.F., PENASSE, L., VANNIER, B., & GLOMOT, R. (1979) Detection of a mutagenic potency of bioallethrin 1/ Microbial assays (2) Micronucleus test in the mouse, Romainville, France, Roussel Uclaf, 36 pp (Unpublished proprietary data).

RICHOLD, M., EDGAR, D.H., RANSOME, S.J., BANKS, S.J., & BOSWORTH, H.J. (1984) An assessment of the mutagenic potential of esbiothrin using an in vitro mammalian cell test system, Huntingdon, United Kingdom, Huntingdon Research Centre, 37 pp (Report No. RSL-EBT-642/84422/A) (Unpublished proprietary data supplied by Roussel Uclaf).

RUIGT, G.S.F. & VAN DEN BERCKEN, J. (1986) Action of pyrethroids on a nerve-muscle preparation of the clawed frog, Xenopus laevis. Pestic. Biochem. Physiol., 25: 176-187.

RUZO, L.O., GAUGHAN, L.C., & CASIDA, J.E. (1980) Pyrethroid photochemistry: S-Bioallethrin. J. agric. food Chem., 28: 246-249.

SAKAMOTO, Y., MATSUMOTO, K., & OGAMI, H. (1975a) Irritant effect of esbiol and allethrin on the eye mucosa of the rabbit, Osaka, Japan, Osaka University Medical School, 4 pp (Report No. OU-SB-75.03.22/A) (Unpublished proprietary data supplied by Roussel Uclaf).

SAKAMOTO, Y., MATSUMOTO, K., & OGAMI, H. (1975b) Esbiol mosquito coils subacute inhalation toxicity tests in the mouse and rat, Osaka, Japan, Osaka University Medical School, 44 pp (Report No. OU-SB-75.06.07/A) (Unpublished proprietary data supplied by Roussel Uclaf).

SAKAMOTO, Y., MATSUMOTO, K., OGAMI, H., YOSHIMURA, M., SHINADA, T., & KAMITAMARI, M. (1975c) Esbiol acute inhalation toxicity tests in the mouse and rat, Osaka, Japan, Osaka University Medical School, 15 pp (Report No. OU-SB-75.02.15/A) (Unpublished proprietary data supplied by Roussel Uclaf).

SAKAMOTO, Y., MATSUMOTO, K., OGAMI, H., YOSHIMURA, M., SANO, N., & SHIMADA, T. (1975d) Esbiol subacute inhalation toxicity tests in the mouse and rat (one-month), Osaka, Japan, Osaka University Medical School, 52 pp (Report No. OU-SB-75.05.27/A) (Unpublished proprietary data supplied by Roussel Uclaf).

SAKAUE, S., DOI, T., & DOI, T. (1985) Determination of allethrin and other pesticides in mosquito coils by the shaking extraction method. Agric. biol. Chem., 49(4): 921-924.

SANDERS, H.J. & TAFF, A.W. (1954) Allethrin. Ind. eng. Chem., 46: 414-426.

SANDERS, H.O. (1969) Toxicity of pesticides to the crustaneans, Gammarus lacustris, Washington, DC, US Department of the Interior, Bureau of Sport Fishery and Wildlife, p. 18 (Technical Paper No. 25).

SANDERS, H.O. & COPE, O.B. (1966) Toxicities of several pesticides to two species of Cladocerans. Trans. Am. Fish. Soc., 95: 165-169.

SANDERS, H.O. & COPE, O.B. (1968) The relative toxicities of several pesticides to naiads of three species of stoneflies. Limnol. Oceanogr., 13: 112-117.

SASAKI, M., SUGIMURA, K., YOSHIDA, A., & ABE, S. (1980) Cytogenetic effects of 60 chemicals on cultured human and Chinese hamster cells. Kromosomo II, 20: 574-584.

SATO, H., ARAI, M., HAGIWARA, A., & ARAI, M. (1985) Chronic toxicity and oncogenicity study of Pynamin Forte in rats, Nagoya, Japan, Daiyu-kai Institute of Medical Sciences (Technical Report No. KT-51-0058) (Proprietary data made available by Sumitomo Chemical Co., Ltd).

SAUNDERS, J.L. & VERCOE, R.R. (1970) Sensitization study with bioallethrin on guinea pigs, Berkhamsted, United Kingdom, Wellcome Foundation Ltd, 4 pp (Report No. WELL-BA-70.23.02/A) (Unpublished proprietary data supplied by Roussel Uclaf).

SCHECHTER, M.S., GREEN, N., & LAFORGE, F.B. (1949) Constituents of pyrethrum flowers XXIII. Cinerolone and synthesis of related cyclopentenolones. J. Am. Chem. Soc., 71: 3165-3173.

SHERBY, S.M., ELDEFRAWI, A.T., DESHPANDE, S.S., ALBUQUERQUE, E.X., & ELDEFRAWI, M.E. (1986) Effects of pyrethroids on nicotinic acetylcholine receptor binding and function. Pestic. Biochem. Physiol., 26: 107-115.

SHINODA, N., SUGIYAMA, O., & TAKAGAKI, Y. (1975) Esbiol teratological test results in rats and mice, Japan, Chugai Pharmaceutical Co., Ltd, 42 pp (Report No. CP-SB-75.02.28.A) (Unpublished proprietary data supplied by Roussel Uclaf).

STARKUS, J.G. & NARAHASHI, T. (1978) Temperature dependence of allethrin-induced repetitive discharges in nerves. Pestic. Biochem. Physiol., 9: 225-230.

STEVENSON, J.H., NEEDHAM, P.H., & WALKER, J. (1978) Poisoning of honey-bee by pesticides: Investigations of the changing pattern in Britain over 20 years, Rothamsted, United Kingdom, Rothamsted Experimental Station, Part 2, pp. 55-72.

SUZUKI, H. (1975) Mutagenicity of some synthetic pyrethroids in bacterial test systems, Takarazuka, Sumitomo Chemical Co., Ltd (Report No. KT-50-0026) (Unpublished proprietary information made available by Sumitomo Chemical Co., Ltd).

SUZUKI, H. (1979) In vitro sister chromatid exchange test of allethrin, Takarazuka, Sumitomo Chemical Co., Ltd (Report No. KT-90-0055) (Unpublished proprietary information made available by Sumitomo Chemical Co., Ltd).

TSUCHIYAMA, H., SUGIHARA, S., KAWAI, K., ITOH, M., MEGURO, H., HARA, N., & KUBO, T. (1975) Electric mosquito mat, subacute inhalation toxicity tests in mice, Nagasaki, Japan, Nagasaki University Medical School, 77 pp (Report No. NU-SB-75.08.24/A) (Unpublished proprietary data supplied by Roussel Uclaf).

TUCKER, R.K. & CRABTREE, D.G. (1970) Handbook of toxicity of pesticides to wildlife, Washington, DC, US Department of the Interior, Bureau of Sport Fishery and Wildlife, 131 pp (Resource Publication No. 84131).

UNO, M., OKADA, T., OHMAE, T., TERADA, I., & TANIGAWA, K. (1982) [Determination of pyrethroid insecticides by dual-wavelength densitometry.] Shokuhin Eiseigaku Zasshi, 23: 191-195 (in Japanese).

VAN DEN BERCKEN, J. (1977) The action of allethrin on the peripheral nervous system of the frog. Pestic. Sci., 8: 692-699.

VAN DEN BERCKEN, J. & VIJVERBERG, H.P.M. (1980) Voltage clamp studies on the effects of allethrin and DDT on the sodium channels in frog myelinated nerve membrane. In: Insect neurobiology and pesticide action (Neutox 79)2, London, Society of Chemical Industry, pp. 78-85.

VAN DEN BERCKEN, J., AKKERMANS, L.M.A., & VAN DER ZALM, J.M. (1973) DDT-like action of allethrin in the sensory nervous system of Xenopus laevis. Eur. J. Pharmacol., 21: 95-106.

VAN DEN BERCKEN, J., KROESE, A.B.A., & AKKERMANS, L.M.A. (1979) Effects of insecticides on the sensory nervous system. In: Narahashi, T., ed. Neurotoxicology of insecticides and pheromones, New York, Plenum Press, pp. 183-210.

VANNIER, B. & FOURNEX, R. (1984) Esbiothrin. Detection of mutagenic potency (micronucleus test in the mouse), Romainville, France, Roussel Uclaf, 14 pp (Report No. RU-EBT-84.603/A) (Unpublished proprietary data).

VERCOE, R.R. & MALONE, J.C. (1969) Dermal irritancy of pyrethroids and piperonyl butoxide to rabbits, Berkhamsted, United Kingdom, Wellcome Foundation Ltd, 5 pp (Report No. WELL-BA-69.19.03/A) (Unpublished proprietary data supplied by Roussel Uclaf).

VERSCHOYLE, R.D. & ALDRIDGE, W.N. (1980) Structure-activity relationship of some pyrethroids in rats. Arch. Toxicol., 45: 325-329.

VERSCHOYLE, R.D. & BARNES, J.M. (1972) Toxicity of natural and synthetic pyrethrins to rats. Pestic. Biochem. Physiol., 2: 308-311.

VIJVERBERG, H.P.M. & VAN DEN BERCKEN, J. (1979) Frequency dependent effects of the pyrethroid insecticide decamethrin in frog myelinated nerve fibres. Eur. J. Pharmacol., 58: 501-504.

VIJVERBERG, H.P.M. & VAN DEN BERCKEN, J. (1982) Action of pyrethroid insecticides on the vertebrate nervous system. Neuropathol. appl. Neurobiol., 8: 421-440.

VIJVERBERG, H.P.M., RUIGT, G.S.F., & VAN DEN BERCKEN, J. (1982a) Structure-related effects of pyrethroid insecticides on the lateral-line sense organ and on peripheral nerves of the clawed frog, Xenopus laevis. Pestic. Biochem. Physiol., 18: 315-324.

VIJVERBERG, H.P.M., VAN DER ZALM, J.M., & VAN DEN BERCKEN, J. (1982b) Similar mode of action of pyrethroids and DDT on sodium channel gating in myelinated nerves. Nature (Lond.), 295: 601-603.

VIJVERBERG, H.P.M., VAN DER ZALM, J.M., VAN KLEEF, R.G.D.M., & VAN DEN BERCKEN, J. (1983) Temperature- and structure-dependent interaction of pyrethroids with the sodium channel in frog node of Ranvier. Biochem. Biophys. Acta, 728: 73-82.

WALLWORK, L. & MALONE, J.C. (1969) Potentiation studies between bioallethrin and piperonyl butoxide, Berkhamsted, United Kingdom, Wellcome Foundation Ltd, 3 pp (Report No. WELL-BA-69.30.12/A) (Unpublished proprietary data supplied by Roussel Uclaf).

WALLWORK, L., CLAMPITT, R.B., & MALONE, J.C. (1972) Bioallethrin rat oral 90-day toxicity study, Berkhamsted, United Kingdom, Wellcome Foundation Ltd, 77 pp (Report No. WELL-BA-75.16-02/A) (Unpublished proprietary data supplied by Roussel Uclaf).

WANG, C.M., NARAHASHI, T., & SCUKA, M. (1972) Mechanism of negative temperature coefficient of nerve-blocking action of allethrin. J. Pharmacol. exp. Ther., 182: 442-453.

WEATHERHOLTZ, W.M. (1972) Teratology study of Pynamin in rabbits. Final report, Vienna, Virginia, Hazleton Laboratory Inc. (Project No. 343-109) (Proprietary data made available by Sumitomo Chemical Co., Ltd).

WHO (1979) WHO Technical Report Series, No. 634 (Safe use of pesticides. Third Report of the WHO Expert Committee on Vector Biology and Control), pp. 18-24.

WHO (1986) The WHO recommended classification of pesticides by hazard and guidelines to classification 1986-87, Geneva, World Health Organization, p. 38 (VBC/86.1, Rev. 1).

WING, K.D. & HAMMOCK B.D. (1979) Stereoselectivity of a radioimmunoassay for the insecticide S-Bioallethrin. Experientia (Basel), 35: 1619-1620.

WORTHING, C.R. & WALKER, S.B. (1983) The pesticide manual, 7th ed., Croydon, British Crop Protection Council, p. 7.

WOUTERS, W. & VAN DEN BERCKEN, J. (1978) Action of pyrethroids. Gen. Pharmacol., 9: 387-398.

YAMAMOTO, I. (1970) Mode of action of pyrethroids, nicotinoids, and rotenoids. Annu. Rev. Entomol., 15: 257-272.

YAMAMOTO, I., UNAI, T., SUZUKI, Y., & KATSUDA, Y. (1976) Preparation, stabilization, and insecticidal activity of cyclodextrin-inclusion compounds of pyrethroids. J. Pestic. Sci., 1: 41-48.

YOSHIOKA, H. (1980) [Chemistry and action of the recent synthetic pyrethroids and their stereoisomers.] J. synth. org. Chem. Jpn, 38: 1151-1162 (in Japanese).

ZITKO, V., CARSON, W.G., & METCALF, C.D. (1977) Toxicity of pyrethroids to juvenile atlantic salmon. Bull. environ. Contam. Toxicol., 18: 35-41.

APPENDIX

On the basis of electrophysiological studies with peripheral nerve preparations of frogs (<u>Xenopus laevis</u>; <u>Rana temporaria</u>, and <u>Rana esculenta</u>), it is possible to distinguish between 2 classes of pyrethroid insecticides: (Type I and Type II). A similar distinction between these 2 classes of pyrethroids has been made on the basis of the symptoms of toxicity in mammals and insects (Van den Bercken et al., 1979; WHO, 1979; Verschoyle & Aldridge, 1980; Glickman & Casida, 1982; Lawrence & Casida, 1982). The same distinction was found in studies on cockroaches by Gammon et al. (1981).

Based on the binding assay on the gamma-aminobutyric acid (GABA) receptor-ionophore complex, synthetic pyrethroids can also be classified into two types: the α-cyano-3-phenoxybenzyl pyrethroids and the non-cyano pyrethroids (Gammon et al., 1982; Gammon & Casida, 1983; Lawrence & Casida, 1983; Lawrence et al., 1985).

<u>Pyrethroids that do not contain an α-cyano group (allethrin, d-phenothrin, permethrin, tetramethrin, cismethrin, and bioresmethrin) (Type I: T-syndrome)</u>

The pyrethroids that do not contain an α-cyano group give rise to pronounced repetitive activity in sense organs and in sensory nerve fibres (Van den Bercken et al., 1973). At room temperature, this repetitive activity usually consists of trains of 3-10 impulses and occasionally up to 25 impulses. Train duration is between 10 and 5 milliseconds.

These compounds also induce pronounced repetitive firing of the presynaptic motor nerve terminal in the neuromuscular junction (Van den Bercken, 1977). There was no significant effect of the insecticide on neurotransmitter release or on the sensitivity of the subsynaptic membrane or the muscle fibre membrane. Presynaptic repetitive firing was also observed in the sympathetic ganglion treated with these pyrethroids.

In the lateral-line sense organ and in the motor nerve terminal, but not in the cutaneous touch receptor or in sensory nerve fibres, the pyrethroid-induced repetitive activity increases dramatically as the temperature is lowered, and a decrease of 5 °C in temperature may cause a more than 3-fold increase in the number of repetitive impulses per train. This effect is easily reversed by raising the temperature. The origin of this "negative temperature coefficient" is not clear (Vijverberg et al., 1983).

Synthetic pyrethroids act directly on the axon through interference with the sodium channel gating mechanism that underlies the generation and conduction of each nerve impulse. The transitional state of the sodium channel is controlled by 2 separately acting gating mechanisms, referred to as the activation gate and the inactivation gate. Since pyrethroids only appear to affect the sodium current during depolarization, the rapid opening of the activation gate and the slow closing of the inactivation gate proceed normally. However, once the sodium channel is open, the activation gate is restrained in the open position by the pyrethroid molecule. While all pyrethroids have essentially the same basic mechanism of action, the rate of relaxation differs substantially for the various pyrethroids (Flannigan & Tucker, 1985).

In the isolated node of Ranvier, allethrin causes prolongation of the transient increase in sodium permeability of the nerve membrane during excitation (Van den Bercken & Vijverberg, 1980). Evidence so far available indicates that allethrin selectively slows down the closing of the activation gate of a fraction of the sodium channels that open during depolarization of the membrane. The time constant of closing of the activation gate in the allethrin-affected channels is about 100 milliseconds compared with less than 100 microseconds in the normal sodium channel, i.e., it is slowed down by a factor of more than 100. This results in a marked prolongation of the sodium current across the nerve membrane during excitation, and this prolonged sodium current is directly responsible for the repetitive activity induced by allethrin (Vijverberg et al., 1983).

The effects of cismethrin on synaptic transmission in the frog neuromuscular junction, as reported by Evans (1976), are almost identical to those of allethrin, i.e., presynaptic repetitive firing, and no significant effects on transmitter release or on the subsynaptic membrane.

Interestingly, the action of these pyrethroids closely resembles that of the insecticide DDT in the peripheral nervous system of the frog. DDT also causes pronounced repetitive activity in sense organs, in sensory nerve fibres, and in motor nerve terminals, due to a prolongation of the transient increase in sodium permeability of the nerve membrane during excitation. Recently, it was demonstrated that allethrin and DDT have essentially the same effect on sodium channels in frog myelinated nerve membrane. Both compounds slow down the rate of closing of a fraction of the sodium channels that open on depolarization of the membrane (Van den Bercken et al., 1973, 1979; Vijverberg et al., 1982b).

In the electrophysiological experiments using giant axons of crayfish, the Type I pyrethroids and DDT analogues retain sodium channels in a modified open state only intermittantly, cause large depolarizing after-potentials, and evoke repetitive firing with minimal effect on the resting potential (Lund & Narahashi, 1983).

These results strongly suggest that permethrin and cismethrin, like allethrin, primarily affect the sodium channels in the nerve membrane and cause a prolongation of the transient increase in sodium permeability of the membrane during excitation.

The effects of pyrethroids on end-plate and muscle action potentials were studied in the pectoralis nerve-muscle preparation of the clawed frog (*Xenopus laevis*). Type I pyrethroids (allethrin, cismethrin, bioresmethrin, and 1R, *cis*-phenothrin) caused moderate presynaptic repetitive activity, resulting in the occurrence of multiple end-plate potentials (Ruigt & Van den Bercken, 1986).

Pyrethroids with an α-cyano group on the 3-phenoxybenzyl alcohol (deltamethrin, cypermethrin, fenvalerate, and fenpropanate) (Type II: CS-syndrome)

The pyrethroids with an α-cyano group cause an intense repetitive activity in the lateral-line organ in the form of long-lasting trains of impulses (Vijverberg et al., 1982a). Such a train may last for up to 1 min and contains thousands of impulses. The duration of the trains and the number of impulses per train increase markedly on lowering the temperature. Cypermethrin does not cause repetitive activity in myelinated nerve fibres. Instead, this pyrethroid causes a frequency-dependent depression of the nervous impulse, brought about by a progressive depolarization of the nerve membrane as a result of the summation of depolarizing after-potentials during train stimulation (Vijverberg & Van den Bercken, 1979; Vijverberg et al., 1983).

In the isolated node of Ranvier, cypermethrin, like allethrin, specifically affects the sodium channels of the nerve membrane and causes a long-lasting prolongation of the transient increase in sodium permeability during excitation, presumably by slowing down the closing of the activation gate of the sodium channel (Vijverberg & Van den Bercken, 1979; Vijverberg et al., 1983). The time constant of closing of the activation gate in the cypermethrin-affected channels is prolonged to more than 100 milliseconds. Apparently, the amplitude of the prolonged sodium current after cypermethrin is too small to induce repetitive activity in nerve fibres, but is sufficient to cause the long-lasting repetitive firing in the lateral-line sense organ.

These results suggest that α-cyano pyrethroids primarily affect the sodium channels in the nerve membrane and cause a long-lasting prolongation of the transient increase in sodium permeability of the membrane during excitation.

In the electrophysiological experiments using giant axons of crayfish, the Type II pyrethroids retain sodium channels in a modified continuous open state persistently, depolarize the membrane, and block the action potential without causing repetitive firing (Lund & Narahashi, 1983).

Diazepam, which facilitates GABA reaction, delayed the onset of action of deltamethrin and fenvalerate, but not permethrin and allethrin, in both the mouse and cockroach. Possible mechanisms of the Type II pyrethroid syndrome include action at the GABA receptor complex or a closely linked class of neuroreceptor (Gammon et al., 1982).

The Type II syndrome of intracerebrally administered pyrethroids closely approximates that of the convulsant picrotoxin (PTX). Deltamethrin inhibits the binding of [^{3}H]-dihydropicrotoxin to rat brain synaptic membranes, whereas the non-toxic R epimer of deltamethrin is inactive. These findings suggest a possible relation between the Type II pyrethroid action and the GABA receptor complex. The stereospecific correlation between the toxicity of Type II pyrethroids and their potency to inhibit the [^{35}S]-TBPS binding was established using a radioligand, [^{35}S]-t-butyl-bicyclophosphoro-thionate [^{35}S]-TBPS. Studies with 37 pyrethroids revealed an absolute correlation, without any false positive or negative, between mouse intracerebral toxicity and in vitro inhibition: all toxic cyano compounds including deltamethrin, [1R,cis]-cypermethrin, [1R,trans]-cypermethrin, and [2S, αS]-fenvalerate were inhibitors, but their non-toxic stereoisomers were not; non-cyano pyrethroids were much less potent or were inactive (Lawrence & Casida, 1983).

In the [^{35}S]-TBPS and [^{3}H]-Ro 5-4864 (a convulsant benzodiazepine radioligand) binding assay, the inhibitory potencies of pyrethroids were closely related to their mammalian toxicities. The most toxic pyrethroids of Type II were the most potent inhibitors of [^{3}H]-Ro 5-4864 specific binding to rat brain membranes. The [^{3}H]-dihydropicrotoxin and [^{35}S]-TBPS binding studies with pyrethroids strongly indicated that Type II effects of pyrethroids are mediated, at least in part, through an interaction with a GABA-regulated chloride ionophore-associated binding site. Moreover, studies with [^{3}H]-Ro 5-4864 support this hypothesis and, in addition, indicate that the pyrethroid-binding site may be very closely related to the convulsant benzodiazepine site of action (Lawrence et al., 1985).

The Type II pyrethroids (deltamethrin, [1R,cis]-cypermethrin and [2S,αS]-fenvalerate) increased the input resistance of crayfish claw opener muscle fibres bathed in GABA. In contrast, two non-insecticidal stereoisomers and Type I pyrethroids (permethrin, resmethrin, allethrin) were inactive. Therefore, cyanophenoxybenzyl pyrethroids appear to act on the GABA receptor-ionophore complex (Gammon & Casida, 1983).

The effects of pyrethroids on end-plate and muscle action potentials were studied in the pectoralis nerve-muscle preparation of the clawed frog (Xenopus laevis). Type II pyrethroids (cypermethrin and deltamethrin) induced trains of repetitive muscle action potentials without presynaptic repetitive activity. However, an intermediate group of pyrethroids (1R-permethrin, cyphenothrin, and fenvalerate) caused both types of effect. Thus, in muscle or nerve membrane, the pyrethroid induced repetitive activities due to a prolongation of the sodium current. But no clear distinction was observed between non-cyano and α-cyano pyrethroids (Ruigt & Van den Bercken, 1986).

Appraisal

In summary, the results strongly suggest that the primary target site of pyrethroid insecticides in the vertebrate nervous system is the sodium channel in the nerve membrane. Pyrethroids without an α-cyano group (allethrin, d-phenothrin, permethrin, and cismethrin) cause a moderate prolongation of the transient increase in sodium permeability of the nerve membrane during excitation. This results in relatively short trains of repetitive nerve impulses in sense organs, sensory (afferent) nerve fibres, and, in effect, nerve terminals. On the other hand, the α-cyano pyrethroids cause a long-lasting prolongation of the transient increase in sodium permeability of the nerve membrane during excitation. This results in long-lasting trains of repetitive impulses in sense organs and a frequency-dependent depression of the nerve impulse in nerve fibres. The difference in effects between permethrin and cypermethrin, which have identical molecular structures except for the presence of an α-cyano group on the phenoxybenzyl alcohol, indicates that it is this α-cyano group that is responsible for the long-lasting prolongation of the sodium permeability.

Since the mechanisms responsible for nerve impulse generation and conduction are basically the same throughout the entire nervous system, pyrethroids may also induce repetitive activity in various parts of the brain. The difference in symptoms of poisoning by α-cyano pyrethroids, compared with the classical pyrethroids, is not necessarily due to an exclusive central site of action. It may be related to the long-lasting repetitive activity in sense organs and possibly in other parts of the nervous system, which, in a more advance state of poisoning, may be accompanied by a frequency-dependent depression of the nervous impulse.

Pyrethroids also cause pronounced repetitive activity and a prolongation of the transient increase in sodium permeability of the nerve membrane in insects and other invertebrates. Available information indicates that the sodium channel in the nerve membrane is also the most important target site of pyrethroids in the invertebrate nervous system (Wouters & Van den Bercken, 1978; WHO, 1979).

Because of the universal character of the processes underlying nerve excitability, the action of pyrethroids should not be considered restricted to particular animal species, or to a certain region of the nervous system. Although it has been established that sense organs and nerve endings are the most vulnerable to the action of pyrethroids, the ultimate lesion that causes death will depend on the animal species, environmental conditions, and on the chemical structure and physical characteristics of the pyrethroid molecule (Vijverberg & Van den Bercken, 1982).

Other titles available in the ENVIRONMENTAL HEALTH CRITERIA series (continued):

44. Mirex
45. Camphechlor
46. Guidelines for the Study of Genetic Effects in Human Populations
47. Summary Report on the Evaluation of Short-Term Tests for Carcinogens (Collaborative Study on *In Vitro* Tests)
48. Dimethyl Sulfate
49. Acrylamide
50. Trichloroethylene
51. Guide to Short-Term Tests for Detecting Mutagenic and Carcinogenic Chemicals
52. Toluene
53. Asbestos and Other Natural Mineral Fibres
54. Ammonia
55. Ethylene Oxide
56. Propylene Oxide
57. Principles of Toxicokinetic Studies
58. Selenium
59. Principles for Evaluating Health Risks from Chemicals During Infancy and Early Childhood: The Need for a Special Approach
60. Principles and Methods for the Assessment of Neurotoxicity Associated With Exposure to Chemicals
61. Chromium
62. 1,2-Dichloroethane
63. Organophosphorus Insecticides — A General Introduction
64. Carbamate Pesticides — A General Introduction
65. Butanols — Four Isomers
66. Kelevan
67. Tetradifon
68. Hydrazine
69. Magnetic Fields
70. Principles for the Safety Assessment of Food Additives and Contaminants in Food
71. Pentachlorophenol
72. Principles of Studies on Diseases of Suspected Chemical Etiology and Their Prevention
73. Phosphine and Selected Metal Phosphides
74. Diaminotoluenes
75. Toluene Diisocyanates
76. Thiocarbamate Pesticides — A General Introduction
77. Man-Made Mineral Fibres
78. Dithiocarbamate Pesticides
79. Dichlorvos
80. Pyrrolizidine Alkaloids
81. Vanadium
82. Cypermethrin
83. DDT and its Derivatives — Environmental Aspects
84. 2,4-Dichlorophenoxyacetic Acid — Environmental Aspects
85. Lead — Environmental Aspects
86. Mercury — Environmental Aspects